English for Rehabilitation Medicine

康复医学英语

主　编　祝亚平
副主编　刘　敏
编　者　徐　欣　曾思良　杨　玥
　　　　王　珊　王苏蒙　张佳钰
　　　　周萍萍　孟　赛

苏州大学出版社
Soochow University Press

图书在版编目(CIP)数据

康复医学英语 = English for Rehabilitation Medicine / 祝亚平主编. —苏州：苏州大学出版社，2022.8（2025.6重印）

ISBN 978-7-5672-3986-9

Ⅰ.①康… Ⅱ.①祝… Ⅲ.①康复医学-英语 Ⅳ.①R49

中国版本图书馆 CIP 数据核字(2022)第 123912 号

书　　名：	康复医学英语 English for Rehabilitation Medicine
主　　编：	祝亚平
责任编辑：	沈　琴
出版发行：	苏州大学出版社（Soochow University Press）
地　　址：	苏州市十梓街 1 号　邮编：215006
印　　装：	苏州市越洋印刷有限公司
网　　址：	http://www.sudapress.com
邮　　箱：	sdcbs@suda.edu.cn
邮购热线：	0512-67480030
销售热线：	0512-67481020
开　　本：	889 mm×1 194mm　1/16　印张：10.25　字数：274 千
版　　次：	2022 年 8 月第 1 版
印　　次：	2025 年 6 月第 2 次印刷
书　　号：	ISBN 978-7-5672-3986-9
定　　价：	58.00 元

凡购本社图书发现印装错误，请与本社联系调换。服务热线：0512-67481020

编者的话

康复医学是近年来发展迅速的医学技术类学科,其发展伴随着越来越频繁而广泛的国际技术交流。因此,从业人员加强专业英语的学习十分必要。当前,全国有百余所院校开设了康复治疗学专业,有些院校开设了康复专业英语,亟须一部适合我国康复医学专业学生使用的专业英语教材。

上海师范大学天华学院于2017年开始与美国威斯康星协和大学合作,联合培养康复治疗学本科生,该项目获得中华人民共和国教育部的审批。为了使学生能够适应美方教师的全英语教学,我们组织编写了这本《康复医学英语》教材,参考了国外主流的《医学术语》的基本内容,针对康复治疗学专业的特点选编了肌肉骨骼、神经和循环系统的解剖生理内容,也选编了康复医学的主要分支如物理治疗、作业治疗、言语康复、儿童康复、精神康复的内容,并且介绍了国际功能、残疾和健康分类(ICF)的基本概念。为了加强学生职业操守的养成,开篇选编了希波克拉底誓言的内容。本教材附有词汇表、练习题,并提供练习题的参考答案,使用者可扫二维码获取。附录选编了常用的医学术语词根与词缀,可以配合36课时的教学实践。5年的教学试用与修改完善形成了这部适用于康复治疗学专业英语教学及康复医学从业者学习的实用教材。通过本教材的学习,学习者可以掌握医学英语的基本术语及康复治疗学专业的基本词汇,达到用英语进行康复专业基本阅读及交流沟通的初级水平。

本教材由祝亚平任主编,刘敏任副主编,徐欣、曾思良、杨玥、王珊、王苏蒙、张佳钰、周萍萍、孟赛参与了编写。本书成稿后得到美国威斯康星协和大学康复治疗系前主任泰德·金博士(Dr. Ted J. King)的审阅并提出了宝贵意见。本教材得以出版,责任编辑沈琴也付出了巨大的努力,在此一并表示感谢!

由于编者水平所限,书中疏漏和不足在所难免,恳请读者不吝赐教。

Contents

■ **CHAPTER 1**
　　HIPPOCRATIC OATH　/ 1

■ **CHAPTER 2**
　　BASIC STRUCTURE OF MEDICAL TERMS　/ 7

■ **CHAPTER 3**
　　BODY SYSTEMS　/ 13

■ **CHAPTER 4**
　　HUMAN GROWTH AND DEVELOPMENT　/ 30

■ **CHAPTER 5**
　　MUSCULOSKELETAL SYSTEM　/ 40

■ **CHAPTER 6**
　　NERVOUS SYSTEM　/ 72

■ **CHAPTER 7**
　　CIRCULATORY SYSTEM　/ 89

■ **CHAPTER 8**
　　THE ICF : AN OVERVIEW　/ 98

■ **CHAPTER 9**
　　PHYSICAL THERAPY　/ 106

■ **CHAPTER 10**
　　OCCUPATIONAL THREAPY　/ 113

■ **CHAPTER 11**
　　SPEECH AND LANGUAGE REHABILITATION　/ 122

■ **CHAPTER 12**
　　PEDIATRIC REHABILITATION　/ 129

■ **CHAPTER 13**
　　PSYCHIATRIC REHABILITATION　/ 135

■ **APPENDIX**　/ 143

CHAPTER 1

HIPPOCRATIC OATH
希波克拉底誓言

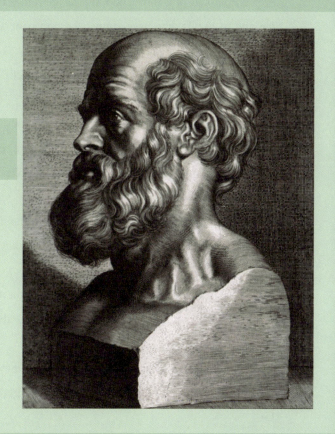

Chapter Sections

Hippocratic Oath: classical version
Hippocratic Oath: modern version
Notes
Vocabulary

Chapter Goals

- To know the content of the classical version of the Hippocratic Oath.
- To briefly describe the meaning of the modern version of the Hippocratic Oath.
- To compare the differences between the two versions.

HIPPOCRATIC OATH: CLASSICAL VERSION

I swear by Apollo the Physician, and Asclepius and Hygieia and Panacea and all the gods and goddesses, making them my witnesses, that I will fulfill according to my ability and judgment this oath and this covenant:

To hold him who has taught me this art as equal to my parents and to live my life in partnership with him, and if he is in need of money to give him a share of mine, and to regard his offspring as equal to my brothers in male lineage and to teach them this art—if they desire to learn it—without fee and covenant; to give a share of precepts and oral instruction and all the other learning to my sons and to the sons of him who has instructed me and to pupils who have signed the covenant and have taken an oath according to the medical law, but no one else.

I will apply dietetic measures for the benefit of the sick according to my ability and judgment; I will keep them from harm and injustice.

I will neither give a deadly drug to anybody who asked for it, nor will I make a suggestion to this effect. Similarly I will not give to a woman an abortive remedy. In purity and holiness I will guard my life and my art.

I will not use the knife, not even on sufferers from stone, but will withdraw in favor of such men as are engaged in this work.

Whatever houses I may visit, I will come for the benefit of the sick, remaining free of all intentional injustice, of all mischief and in particular of sexual relations with both female and male persons, be they free or slaves.

What I may see or hear in the course of the treatment or even outside of the treatment in regard to the life of men, which on no account one must spread abroad, I will keep to myself, holding such things shameful to be spoken about.

If I fulfill this oath and do not violate it, may it be granted to me to enjoy life and art, being honored with fame among all men for all time to come; if I transgress it and swear falsely, may the opposite of all this be my lot.

—Translation from the Greek by Ludwig Edelstein. From *The Hippocratic Oath: Text, Translation, and Interpretation*, by Ludwig Edelstein. Baltimore: Johns Hopkins Press, 1943.

HIPPOCRATIC OATH: MODERN VERSION

I swear to fulfill, to the best of my ability and judgment, this covenant:

I will respect the hard-won scientific gains of those physicians in whose steps I walk, and gladly share such knowledge as is mine with those who are to follow.

I will apply, for the benefit of the sick, all measures [that] are required, avoiding those twin traps of overtreatment and therapeutic nihilism.

I will remember that there is art to medicine as well as science, and that warmth, sympathy, and understanding may outweigh the surgeon's knife or the chemist's drug.

I will not be ashamed to say "I know not", nor will I fail to call in my colleagues when the skills of another are needed for a patient's recovery.

I will respect the privacy of my patients, for their problems are not disclosed to me that the world may know. Most especially must I tread with care in matters of life and death. If it is given me to save a life, all thanks. But it may also be within my power to take a life; this awesome responsibility must be faced with great humbleness and awareness of my own frailty. Above all, I must not play at God.

I will remember that I do not treat a fever chart, a cancerous growth, but a sick human being, whose illness may affect the person's family and economic stability. My responsibility includes these related problems, if I am to care adequately for the sick.

I will prevent disease whenever I can, for prevention is preferable to cure.

I will remember that I remain a member of society, with special obligations to all my fellow human beings, those sound of mind and body as well as the infirm.

If I do not violate this oath, may I enjoy life and art, respected while I live and remembered with affection thereafter. May I always act so as to preserve the finest traditions of my calling and may I long experience the joy of healing those who seek my help.

—Written in 1964 by Louis Lasagna, Academic Dean of the School of Medicine at Tufts University, and used in many medical schools today.

NOTES

1. Hippocrates: Also called Hippocrates of Cos or Hippokrates of Kos, a medicine and author of the Hippocratic Oath. A collection of around seventy early medical works from ancient Greece was attributed to him, which were collected in the *Hippocratic Collection* (*Corpus Hippocraticum*).

2. Apollo: one of the most important and complex of the Olympian deities in classical Greek and Roman religion and mythology.

3. Asclepius: a hero and god of medicine in ancient Greek religion and mythology.

4. Hygieia: the Goddess of good health, cleanliness, and sanitation.

5. Panacea: In Greek mythology, Panacea was a goddess of universal remedy and the daughter of Asclepius and Epione.

Vocabulary

单词	音标	词性	释义
oath	/əʊθ/	n.	誓言,誓约;诅咒,咒骂
swear	/sweə(r)/	vt.	郑重承诺,发誓要,表示决心要
witness	/ˈwɪtnəs/	n. vt.	目击者,见证人;证人;见证(以言行证实信仰) 当场看到,目击;证明……真实,为……提供证据;见证
fulfill	/fʊlˈfɪl/	vt.	履行;实现;起……作用;使高兴,使满意
judgment	/ˈdʒʌdʒmənt/	n.	判断;裁判;判决书;辨别力
covenant	/ˈkʌvənənt/	n. vt.	承诺;合同;协约;(尤指定期付款的)契约 立约承诺缔结盟约;订协定
offspring	/ˈɒfsprɪŋ/	n.	子女,后代;崽兽;幼崽;幼苗
lineage	/ˈlɪniɪdʒ/	n.	世系;宗系;家系;血统
precept	/ˈpriːsept/	n.	(思想、行为的)准则,规范
oral	/ˈɔːrəl, ˈɒ-/	adj.	口头的;口腔的;口服的
pupil	/ˈpjuːpl/	n.	学生,(尤指)小学生;弟子,门徒;瞳孔
dietetic	/ˌdaɪəˈtetɪk/	adj.	饮食的;营养的
injustice	/ɪnˈdʒʌstɪs/	n.	不公正;不公平(的对待或行为)
abortive	/əˈbɔːtɪv/	adj.	失败的;流产的;堕胎的
remedy	/ˈremədi/	n. vt.	改进措施;补偿;治疗,疗法;药品 改正;纠正;改进
purity	/ˈpjʊərəti/	n.	纯洁;纯净;纯粹
holiness	/ˈhəʊlinəs/	n.	神圣;(对罗马教皇的尊称)圣座
sufferer	/ˈsʌfərə(r)/	n.	患病者;受苦者;受难者
withdraw	/wɪðˈdrɔː, wɪθˈd-/	vt. vi.	使撤回;停止提供;不再给予;使退出;提取(银行账户中的款) 撤回;撤离
intentional	/ɪnˈtenʃnl/	adj.	故意的;有意的;存心的
mischief	/ˈmɪstʃɪf/	n.	顽皮,淘气,恶作剧;恶意,使坏的念头;伤害,毁损
violate	/ˈvaɪəleɪt/	vt.	违反,违犯;侵犯(隐私等);使不得安宁;亵渎,污损(神圣之地)
transgress	/trænzˈgres, træns-/	vt.	越轨;违背(道德);违犯(法律)
overtreatment	/ˌəʊvəˈtriːtmənt/	n.	过度治疗
therapeutic	/ˌθerəˈpjuːtɪk/	adj.	治疗(学)的,医疗的;治病的

nihilism	/ˈnaɪəˌlɪzəm, ˈnaɪɪlɪzəm/	n.	虚无主义
sympathy	/ˈsɪmpəθi/	n.	同情;赞同,支持;意气相投
disclose	/dɪsˈkləʊz/	vt.	揭露;透露;泄露
tread	/tred/	vi. vt. n.	踏;踩;践踏 践踏,踩碎;行走 步法,步态,脚步声;外胎花纹
humbleness	/ˈhʌmblnəs/	n.	谦逊,虚心;低下,卑微
frailty	/ˈfreɪlti/	n.	虚弱;弱点
cancerous	/ˈkænsərəs/	adj.	癌的;像癌的;得癌症的
obligation	/ˌɒblɪˈɡeɪʃn/	n.	义务,责任;证券,契约;债务;恩惠
thereafter	/ˌðeərˈɑːftə(r)/	adv.	之后;此后;以后
preserve	/prɪˈzɜːv/	vt.	保护,维护;保存,保养;贮存,保鲜

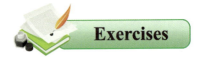

Translate the modern version of the Hippocratic Oath into Chinese.

CHAPTER 2

BASIC STRUCTURE OF MEDICAL TERMS
医学术语的基本结构

Chapter Sections

- Overview
- Origins
- Roots
- Prefixes
- Suffixes
- Combining forms
- Exercises

Chapter Goals

- To identify basic objectives to guide your study of the medical language.
- To divide medical words into their component parts.
- To learn the meaning of basic combining forms, suffixes, and prefixes of the medical language.
- To use these combining forms, suffixes, and prefixes to build medical vocabulary.

OVERVIEW

Medicine has a language of its own. The medical language, like the general language of human beings, possesses a historical development. Current medical vocabulary includes terms used by Hippocrates and Aristotle more than 2,000 years ago, eponyms (words based on or derived from the personal names of people), and terms from modern language. With the advancement of medical and scientific knowledge, medical language changes, discarding some words, altering the meaning of others, and adding new words.

Still, the majority of medical terms in current use are composed of Greek and Latin word parts that maintain the same meaning wherever they appear, which makes it possible to learn the medical language by learning these word parts. Learning word parts and how they fit together to form medical terms provides the key to learning and remembering a wealth of medical vocabulary.

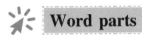

Word parts

Word components fall into three categories:

1. The root is the fundamental unit of each word. It establishes the basic meaning of the word and is the part to which modifying word parts are added.

2. A prefix is a short word part added before a root to modify its meaning. This book indicates prefixes by a dash after the prefix, such as pre-(before).

3. A suffix is a short word part or series of parts added at the end of a root to modify its meaning. This book indicates suffixes by a dash before the suffix, such as -itis (inflammation).

ORIGINS

Medical terminology has a long and rich history that evolved in great measure from the Latin and Greek languages. It is estimated that about three-fourths of our medical terminology is of Greek origin. Latin accounts for the majority of root words in the English language. We find that the oldest written sources of western medicine are the Hippocratic writings from the 5th and 4th centuries BC, which cover all aspects of medicine at that time and contain numerous medical terms. This was the beginning of the Greek era of the language of medicine, which lasted even after the Roman conquest, since the Romans, who had no similar medical tradition, imported Greek medicine. Most of the doctors practicing in the Roman Empire were Greek.

The main reason for this is that the Greeks were the founders of rational medicine in the golden age of

Greek civilization in the 5th century BC. The Hippocratic School and, later on, Galen formulated the theories which dominated medicine up to the beginning of the 18th century. The Hippocratic were the first to describe diseases based on observation, and the names given by them to many conditions are still used today.

A second reason for the large number of Greek medical terms is that the Greek language lends itself easily to the building of compounds. When new terms were needed, with the rapid expansion of medical science during the last century, Greek words or Latin words with Greek endings were used to express the new ideas, conditions, or instruments. The new words follow the older models so closely that it is impossible to distinguish the two by their forms. The fact is that about one-half of our medical terminology is less than a century old.

A third reason for using the classical roots is that they form an international language, easily understood by anyone familiar with the subject matter. The Greek terms came into the English language through the Latin. In adapting the Greek words, the Romans used the Latin alphabet. As Romans conquered the then known world, Latin became the universal language of Italy and the provinces. Many centuries after the fall of Rome, Latin still ruled supreme. To this very day, Latin is the language of the Catholic Church, and during the formative period of the western European languages it was incorporated in every one of them. The Romance language, and especially French, is modern Latin, preserving most of the form and spirit of the ancient language. English is to some extent Germanic in form and part of its vocabulary is Germanic, but a considerable section is of Latin ancestry borrowed from the French. Most of the common roots of speech are Anglo-Saxon, but the moment we leave primitive life and advance to more civilized living, our words immediately become Latin. We walk, start, stop, breathe, sleep, wake, talk, live, and lie in Anglo-Saxon but we advance, retreat, approach, retire, inspire, confer, discuss, compare, refute, debate, perish, survive in Latin, and the predominant part of the vocabulary of business, commerce, finance, government, diplomacy, and the sciences is Latin. Greek medicine migrated to Rome at an early date, and many Latin terms crept into its terminology. Latin was the language of science up to the beginning of the 18th Century, so all medical texts were written in Latin. Under the influence of the great anatomical work of Andreas Vesalius, *De humani corporis fabrica* (1543), the terminology of anatomy is almost exclusively Latin. During the Renaissance period, the science of anatomy was begun. Many early anatomists were faculty members in Italian schools of medicine. These early anatomists assigned Latin names to structures that they discovered. This tradition has continued.

ROOTS

Each body system has a set of word roots. For example, many terms used to describe the cardiovascular system (the heart and blood vessels) derive from the roots *cardi-* (heart) and *angi-* (vessel).

Many terms relating to the respiratory system (the lungs and airways) use the roots *pneum-* (air or lung), *pulmon-* (lung), or *bronch-* (airway).

Many words related to the nervous system (the brain, spinal cord, and nerves) are formed from roots *neur-* (nerve) or *cerebr-* (brain).

PREFIXES

A prefix is a word part attached to the beginning of a root to modify its meaning. For example, the word "gastric" means pertaining to the stomach. Adding the prefix *epi-* forms "epigastric", which means pertaining to above the stomach. Adding the prefix *sub-* forms "subgastric", which means pertaining to under the stomach.

Prefixes often give an indication of direction, location, number of parts, time, or orientation. For example, the word lateral means "side". Adding the prefix *uni-*, meaning "one", forms "unilateral", which means "affecting" or "involving one side". Adding the prefix *contra-*, meaning "against" or "opposite", forms "contralateral", which refers to an opposite side. The term "equilateral" means "having equal sides". Prefixes in this book are followed by hyphens to show that word parts are added to the prefix to form a word.

SUFFIXES

A suffix is a word part attached to the end of the root to make the word a noun, a verb or an adjective and often determines how the definition of the word will begin. For example, by using the root *cephal*, meaning the head, the adjective suffix *-ic* forms the word "cephalic", which means pertaining to the head. By adding the suffix *-ocele*, it produces another word "cephalocele", which is the protrusion of a part of the brain through an opening in the skull.

In medical language there are two types of suffixes: simple and compound. Simple suffixes are those suffixes that have nothing added to them, for instance, *-al* in "dental". Compound suffixes, however, are usually formed by joining a root and a simple suffix. For example, the root *log* and the suffix *-y* join to make the compound suffix *-logy*, which means the act or process of studying. The root *scler* and the suffix *-osis* are combined into another compound suffix *-sclerosis*, meaning hardening. The compound suffix *-ectomy* is the combination of a prefix (*ec-*), a root (*tom*), and a suffix (*-y*). It means the process of cutting out or excision.

The suffixes given in this chapter are general ones that are used throughout medical terminology. Additional suffixes will be presented in later chapters, as they pertain to specific body systems.

COMBINING FORMS

Most of the roots, prefixes and suffixes are combining forms in New Latin and hence international scientific vocabulary. There are a few general rules about how they combine (Figure 2-1). First, prefixes and suffixes, most of which are derived from ancient Greek or classical Latin, have a droppable *-o-*. As a general rule, this *-o-* almost always acts as a joint-stem to connect two consonantal roots, e. g. *arthr- + -o- + logy = arthrology*. But generally, the *-o-* is dropped when connecting to a vowel-stem, e. g. *arthr- + itis = arthritis*, instead of * *arthr-o-itis*. Second, medical roots generally go together according to language, i. e. Greek prefixes occur with Greek suffixes and Latin prefixes with Latin suffixes. Although international scientific vocabulary is not stringent about segregating combining forms of different languages, it is advisable when coining new words not to mix different lingual roots.

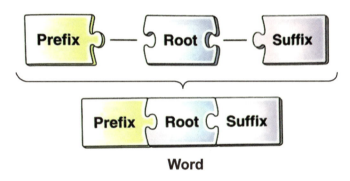

Figure 2-1 Cambining Forms

The Appendix of this book contains lists of different root classification (e. g. body components, quantity, description, etc.). Each list is alphabetized with English meanings and the corresponding Greek and Latin roots given.

Exercises

I *Define the following words.*
1. perioral ___
2. suprapubic ___
3. infraumbilical ___
4. sublingual ___
5. retroperitoneal ___
6. bipedal ___

II *Name the part of the body referred to in the following adjectives.*
1. lumbar ___
2. carpal ___
3. popliteal ___

4. occipital _____
5. phalangeal _____
6. cervical _____
7. celiac _____
8. brachial _____

III *Write a word that means the opposite of each of the following.*
1. infrapatellar _____
2. intracellular _____
3. subscapular _____
4. extrathoracic _____

IV *Write a word that means the same as each of the following.*
1. perioral _____
2. subscapular _____
3. perivascular _____
4. infracostal _____
5. circumorbital _____

CHAPTER 3

BODY SYSTEMS
人体系统

Chapter Sections

- Positional and directional terms
- Planes of the body
- Body cavities
- Abdominopelvic regions and quadrants
- Divisions of the back (Spinal column)
- Body systems
- Terminology
- Exercises

Chapter Goals

- To become acquainted with terms that describe positions and directions.
- To describe division of the body along three different planes.
- To locate and name the nine divisions of the abdomen.
- To locate and name the four quadrants of the abdomen.
- To understand the nine major systems of the human body.

POSITIONAL AND DIRECTIONAL TERMS

When we start to talk about the body, we usually begin with the anatomic position. The body is erected, with the palms of the hands facing outward and the fifth (little) finger in a medial position (closer to the center of the body). The thumb is lateral. This is so called anatomic position. Figure 3-1 shows the positional and directional terms.

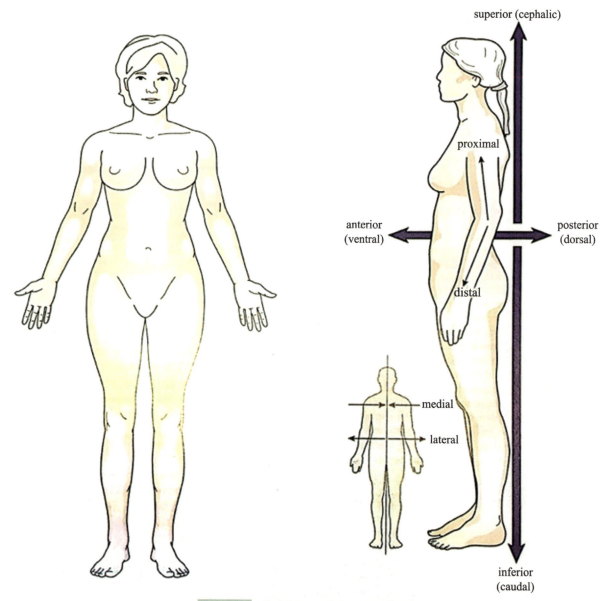

Figure 3-1 Positional and Directional Terms

Table 3-1 identifies the positional and directional terms.

Table 3-1 Positional and Directional Terms

LOCATION	DIRECTION	EXAMPLE
Anterior or ventral	Toward the front; away from the back of the body	The nose is on the anterior side of the face; the toes are anterior to the ankle.
Posterior or dorsal	Near the back; toward the back of the body	The spine is on the posterior side of the body.
Superior or cephalic	Above; toward the head	The neck is superior to the chest.
Inferior or caudal	Below; toward the soles of the feet	The knee is inferior to the hip; the stomach is inferior to the chest.
Proximal	Near the point of attachment to the trunk	The elbow is proximal to the wrist.
Distal	Farther from the point of attachment to the trunk	The fingers are distal to the wrist.
Lateral	Pertaining to the side; away from the middle	The eyes are lateral to the nose.
Medial	Toward the middle of the body	The nose is medial to the eyes.
Prone	Lying horizontal and face down (or turned to the side)	A patient lies on his stomach in the prone position.
Supine	Lying horizontal and face up	The patient was placed on the operating table in a supine position.

PLANES OF THE BODY

A plane is an imaginary flat surface. There are three planes of the body that are frequently used to locate structures or may be used for diagnostic testing. Table 3-2 identifies the planes of the body.

Table 3-2　Planes of the Body

PLANE	LOCATION
Frontal (coronal) plane	**The vertical plane dividing the body or structure into anterior and posterior portions.** A common chest X-ray view is a PA (posteroanterior-viewed from back to front) view, which is in the frontal (coronal) plane.
Sagittal (lateral) plane	**The lengthwise vertical plane dividing the body or structure into right and left sides.** The midsagittal plane divides the body into right and left halves. A lateral (side-to-side) chest X-ray film is taken in the sagittal plane.
Transverse (horizontal) plane	**The horizontal (cross-sectional) plane running across the body parallel to the ground.** This cross-sectional plane divides the body or structure into upper and lower portions. A CT (computed tomography) scan is one of a series of X-ray pictures taken in the transverse (horizontal or cross-sectional) plane.

Figure 3-2 illustrates the planes of the body.

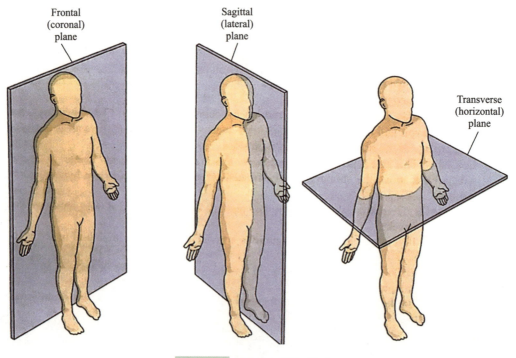

Figure 3-2　Planes of the Body

BODY CAVITIES

Internal organs are located within dorsal and ventral cavities. The dorsal cavity contains the brain in the cranial cavity and the spinal cord in the **spinal cavity**. The uppermost ventral space, the thoracic cavity, is separated from the **abdominal cavity** by the diaphragm, a muscle used in breathing. There is no anatomic separation between the abdominal cavity and the pelvic cavity, which together make up the abdominopelvic cavity (Figure 3-3).

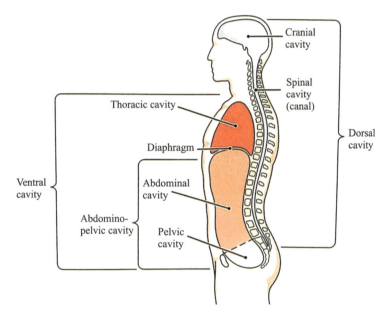

Figure 3-3 Body Cavities (lateral view, shown are the dosal and ventral cavities with their subdivisions)

ABDOMINOPELVIC REGIONS AND QUADRANTS

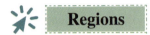 **Regions**

Doctors divide the abdominopelvic area into nine regions (Table 3-3 and Figure 3-4).

Table 3-3 Nine Regions of the Abdominopelvic Cavity

REGIONS	LOCATION
Left hypochondriac region	Left lateral region just below the ribs
Left lumbar region	Left lateral region in the middle row
Left inguinal region	Left lower region of the lower row by the groin
Epigastric region	Middle region in the upper row
Umbilical region	Middle region in the middle row
Hypogastric region	Middle region in the lower row
Right hypochondriac region	Right lateral region just below the ribs
Right lumbar region	Right lateral region in the middle row
Right inguinal region	Right lower region of the lower row by the groin

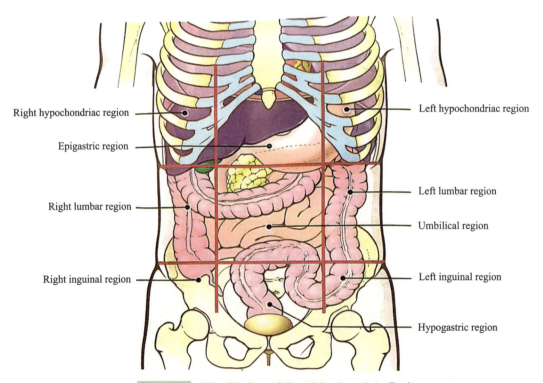

Figure 3-4 Nine Regions of the Abdominopelvic Cavity

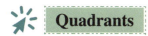 **Quadrants**

The abdominopelvic area can be divided into four quadrants by two imaginary lines—one horizontal and one vertical—that cross at the midsection of the body. Table 3-4 and Figure 3-5 show the four quadrants of the abdominopelvic cavity.

Table 3-4   Four Quadrants of the Abdominopelvic Cavity

QUADRANTS	ORGANS IN QUADRANT
Left upper quadrant (LUQ)	Left lobe of liver, spleen, stomach, portions of the pancreas, portions of small intestines and colon, left kidney
Right upper quadrant (RUQ)	Right lobe of liver, gallbladder, portions of the pancreas, portions of small intestines and colon, right kidney
Right lower quadrant (RLQ)	Portions of small intestines and colon, right ovary and fallopian tube, appendix, and right ureter
Left lower quadrant (LLQ)	Portions of small intestines and colon, left ovary and fallopian tube, and left ureter

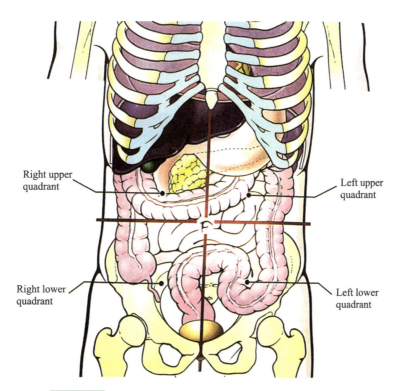

Figure 3-5   Four Quadrants of the Abdominopelvic Cavity

DIVISIONS OF THE BACK (SPINAL COLUMN)

The back (spinal column) is composed of a series of bones that extend from the neck to the coccyx. Each bone is a **vertebra** (plural: vertebrae). Table 3-5 and Figure 3-6 show the divisions of the back. Figure 3-7 shows the MRI (magnetic resonance imaging) of a herniated disk at the L4 – L5 level of the spinal column.

Table 3-5 Divisions of the Back

DIVISION	ABBREVIATION	LOCATION
Cervical	C	Neck region. There are seven cervical vertebrae (C1 to C7).
Thoracic	T	Chest region. There are twelve thoracic vertebrae (T1 to T12). Each bone is joined to a rib.
Lumbar	L	Loin (waist) or flank region (between the ribs and the hipbone). There are five lumbar vertebrae (L1 to L5).
Sacral	S	Five bones (S1 to S5) are fused to form one bone, the sacrum.
Coccygeal	Cy	The coccyx (tailbone) is a small bone composed of four fused pieces.

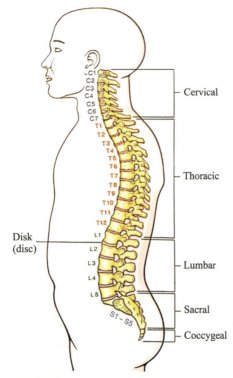

Figure 3-6 Anatomic Divisions of the Back (spinal column)

Note: A disk (disc) is a small pad of cartilage between each backbone.

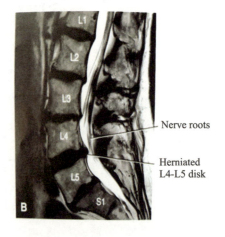

Figure 3-7 MRI of a Herniated Disk at the L4 – L5 Level of the Spinal Column

BODY SYSTEMS

The Human body can be divided to many systems. The musculoskeletal system, the nervous system and the circulatory system are considered most relevant to rehabilitation medicine, so they are explained further in Chapters 5, 6 and 7. The other systems are illustrated with chats below (Figures 3-8, 3-9, 3-10, 3-11, 3-12, 3-13, 3-14).

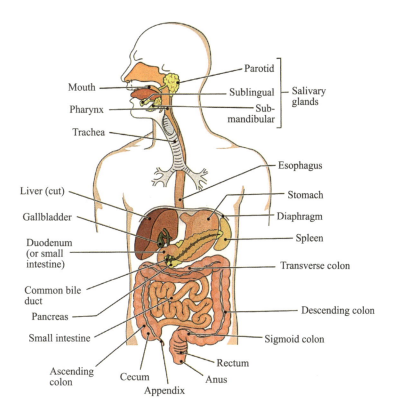

Figure 3-8 Digestive System

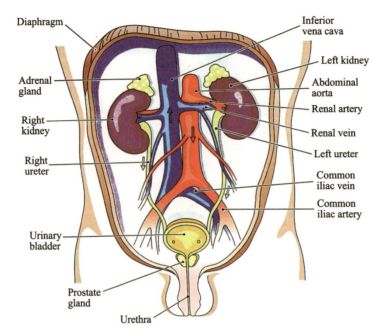

Figure 3-9　Urinary System (male)

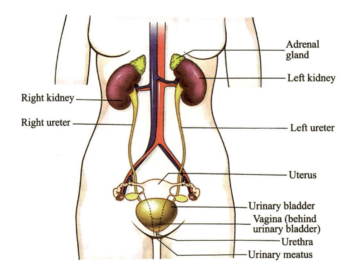

Figure 3-10　Urinary System (female)

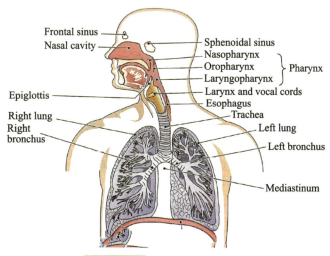

Figure 3-11 Respiratory System

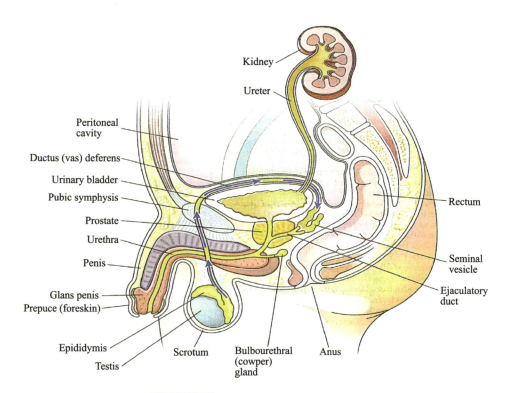

Figure 3-12 Reproductive System (male)

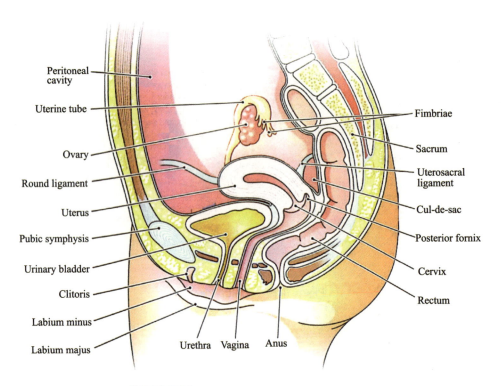

Figure 3-13　Reproductive System(female)

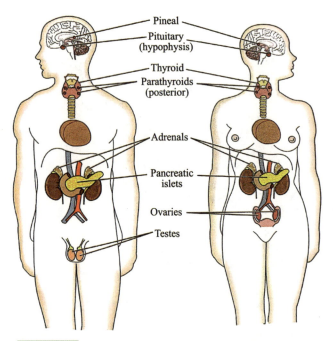

Figure 3-14　Endocrine System(left: male; right: female)

Table 3-6 identifies the body systems.

Table 3-6 Body Systems

SYSTEMS	ORGANS
Digestive system	Mouth, pharynx (throat), esophagus, stomach, intestines (small and large), liver, gallbladder, pancreas
Urinary system	Kidneys, ureters (tubes from the kidneys to the urinary bladder), urinary bladder, urethra (tube from the urinary bladder to the outside of the body)
Respiratory system	Nose, pharynx, larynx (voice box), trachea (windpipe), bronchi, lungs (where the exchange of gases takes place)
Reproductive system	Female: Ovaries, fallopian tubes, uterus (womb), vagina, mammary glands; Male: Testes and associated tubes, urethra, penis, prostate gland
Endocrine system	Thyroid gland (in the neck), pituitary gland (at the base of the brain), sex glands (ovaries and testes), adrenal glands, pancreas (islets of langerhans), parathyroid glands
Nervous system	Brain, spinal cord, nerves, and collections of nerves
Circulatory system	Heart, blood vessels (arteries, veins, and capillaries), lymphatic vessels and nodes, spleen, thymus gland
Musculoskeletal system	Muscles, bones, and joints
Skin and sense organs	Skin, hair, nails, sweat glands, and sebaceous (oil) glands; eye, ear, nose, and tongue

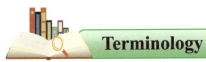

Terminology

Practice spelling each term in Table 3-7 and know its meaning.

Table 3-7 Terminology and Definition

TERMINOLOGY	DEFINITION
Anterior	Toward the front of the body
Posterior	Toward the back of the body
Superior	Toward the head or above something
Inferior	Toward the feet or bellow something
Palmar	Located on, or pertaining to the palm of the hand
Sagittal plane	Any vertical plane that is parallel to the median plane
Frontal plane	A plane that separates the body into anterior and posterior parts
Transverse plane	A plane that divides the body into superior and inferior portions

continued

TERMINOLOGY	DEFINITION
Supine	Lying horizontal and face up
Ventral	Pertaining to, directed towards, or situated on the anterior surface of the body
Dorsal	The back of the body or back of a body part, or positioned more towards the back than some other object or reference
Caudal	Situated towards the lower part of the body
Cavity	A hollow space within the body
Spinal cavity	The space located within the vertebral canal
Ventral cavity	The cavity located along the anterior aspect of the body
Pelvic cavity	The space formed by the hip bones
Hypochondriac	Upper portion of the abdomen, just below the lowest ribs
Epigastric	Above the stomach
Lumbar	Of or near the lower back, between the lowest ribs and pelvis
Umbilical	The navel
Hypogastric	Below (hypo) the stomach area
Digestive system	The set of organs in your body that digest the food you eat
Urinary system	The system that includes all organs involved in reproduction and in the formation and voidance of urine
Respiratory system	The system for taking in oxygen and giving off carbon dioxide, in terrestrial animals this is accomplished by breathing
Reproductive system	Organs and tissues involved in the production and maturation of gametes and in their union and subsequent development as offspring
Endocrine system	The system of glands that produce endocrine secretions that help control bodily metabolic activity
Nervous system	The system that consists of all the nerves in your body together with your brain and spinal cord
Circulatory system	The organs and tissues involved in circulating blood and lymph through the body
Musculoskeletal system	The system relating to muscles and skeleton

CHAPTER 3 BODY SYSTEMS

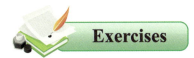 **Exercises**

I *Label the regions and quadrants (use abbreviations) of the abdominopelvic cavity.*

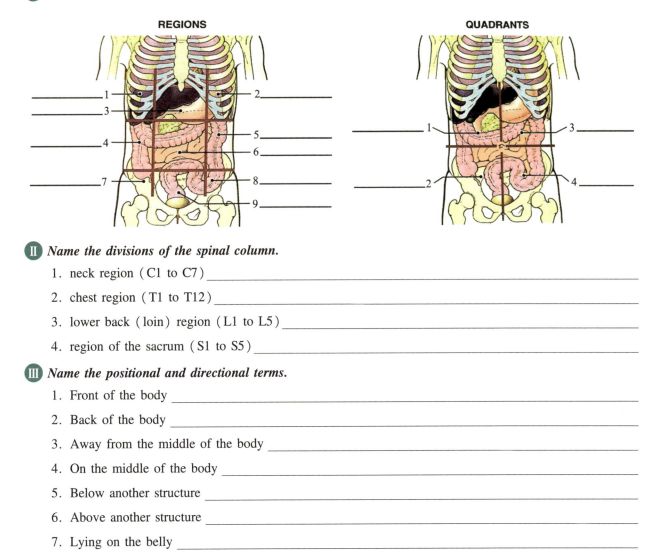

II *Name the divisions of the spinal column.*

1. neck region (C1 to C7) _____

2. chest region (T1 to T12) _____

3. lower back (loin) region (L1 to L5) _____

4. region of the sacrum (S1 to S5) _____

III *Name the positional and directional terms.*

1. Front of the body _____

2. Back of the body _____

3. Away from the middle of the body _____

4. On the middle of the body _____

5. Below another structure _____

6. Above another structure _____

7. Lying on the belly _____

IV *Name the planes of the body as pictured below.*

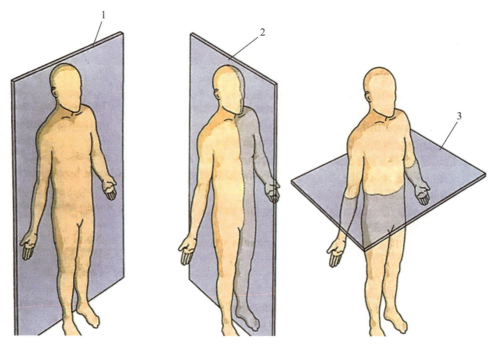

1. _____
2. _____
3. _____

V *The listed terms are planes or quadrants of the body. Match each term with its correct meaning.*

| Frontal (coronal) plane | Right upper quadrant (RUQ) |
| Sagittal (lateral) plane | Transverse (horizontal) plane |

1. Vertical plane that divides the body into anterior and posterior portions: _____

2. Horizontal plane that divides the body into upper and lower portions: _____

3. The section that contains the liver (right lobe), gallbladder, part of the pancreas, parts of the small and large intestines, right kidney: _____

4. Vertical plane that divides the body into right and left portions: _____

VI *Write the major systems of the human body through the given organs.*

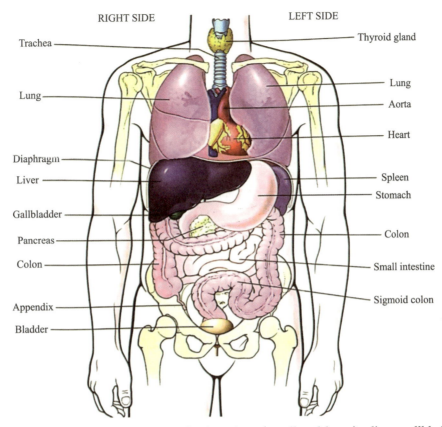

1. Mouth, pharynx (throat), esophagus, stomach, intestines (small and large), liver, gallbladder, pancreas: _____

2. Kidneys, ureters (tubes from the kidneys to the urinary bladder), urinary bladder, urethra (tube from the bladder to the outside of the body): _____

3. Nose, pharynx, larynx (voice box), trachea (windpipe), bronchi, lungs (where the exchange of gases takes place): _____

4. Female: Ovaries, fallopian tubes, uterus (womb), vagina, mammary glands;
   Male: Testes and associated tubes, urethra, penis, prostate gland: _____

5. Brain, spinal cord, nerves, and collections of nerves: _____

CHAPTER 4

HUMAN GROWTH AND DEVELOPMENT
人体生长和发育

Chapter Sections

Introduction

Process of growth and development

Human embryonic and foetal development

The development and configuration of a zygote

Neurologic and psychologic development after birth

A brief introduction of common hypoevolutism happening during infancy

In person: a late developer

Reading: briefing the whole life span

Vocabulary

Exercises

Chapter Goals

- To learn the process about human growth and development from the time of fertilization to the end of infancy.
- To define all the stages during the process.
- To describe neurologic and psychologic development after birth.
- To apply your new knowledge to understanding medical terms in their proper contexts.

INTRODUCTION

Human growth and development is a process of growth and change that takes place between birth and maturity. The process of human growth and development, which takes almost 20 years to complete, is a complex phenomenon. It is under the control of both genetic and environmental influences, which operate in such a way that, at specific times during the period of growth, one or the other may be the dominant influence. The genetic blueprint that includes one's potential for achieving a particular adult size and shape is obtained at the time of conception.

In this chapter, we mainly focus on introducing the things happening from the time of fertilization to the end of infancy while briefly introducing the problems and diseases happening during infancy that require rehabilitation.

PROCESS OF GROWTH AND DEVELOPMENT

1. Definition
   ① Growth is the volume and size increasing of body and organs.
   ② Development are functional maturation of tissues and organs. That is the concept of ongoing change and maturation.
   — Child development encompasses all aspects of pediatrics.
   — It applies to somatic, psychological, and cognitive growth and to behavior.
2. Determinants of growth and development
   — Heredity: the most important factor.
   — Environmental factors (can be improved potentially).
   — Nutrition: an important factor at childhood; the smaller the children's age, the more important.
   — Diseases: a factor that can not be neglected.
   — Seasonality: growth rate varied during the four seasons.
   — Hormone: a complex system.
3. Regular rule of growth & development
   — Upper to lower.
   — Proximal to distal.
   — Rough to fine.
   — Inferior to superior.
   — Simple to complication.

HUMAN EMBRYONIC AND FOETAL DEVELOPMENT

Human embryogenesis refers to the formation and development of the human embryo. It is characterized by the process of cellular differentiation and cell division of the embryo that occurs during the early stages of foetus development.

In biological terms, human development entails its growth from a one-celled zygote to an adult human being. Fertilization occurs when the sperm cell successfully enters and fuses with an egg cell (ovum). The genetic material of the sperm and the egg then combine to form a single cell called a zygote and the germinal stage of prenatal development commences. Embryogenesis covers the first eight weeks of development. At the beginning of the ninth week the embryo is termed a foetus. By the end of the third month, all the organs were basically grown, but without attention, abortion still could occur. After the fifth month, it is safer. Figure 4-1 shows human embryonic and foetal development from the stage of a fertilized egg to a 20 weeks old foetus. And after 20 weeks, the foetus can be examined for the existence of malformation.

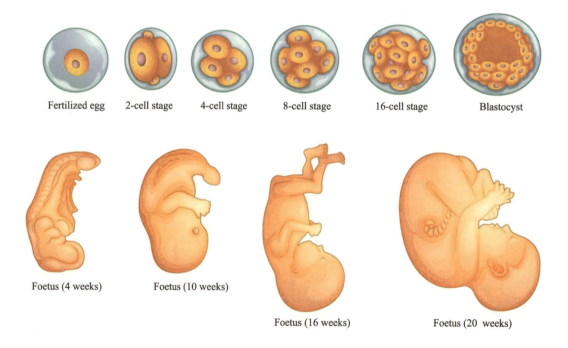

Figure 4-1　Human Embryonic and Foetal Development

THE DEVELOPMENT AND CONFIGURATION OF A ZYGOTE

Zygote refers to the cell resulting from union of a male and female gamete, more precisely, the cell after synapsis at the completion of fertilization until first cleavage. Figure 4-2 shows the previous development of the zygote.

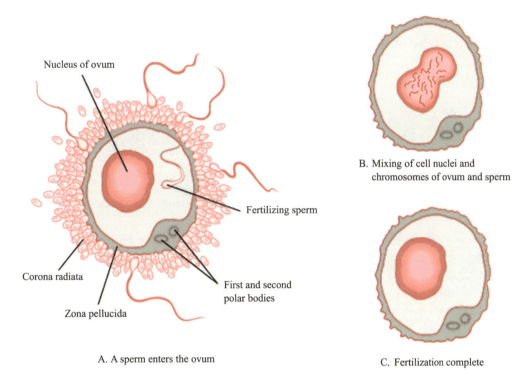

Figure 4-2 **Previous Development of the Zygote**

A: A sperm enters the ovum. B: The 23 chromosomes from the sperm mingle with the 23 chromosomes from the ovum, restoring the diploid number to 46. C: The fertilized ovum, now called a zygote, is ready for the first mitotic cell division.

After fertilization, the conceptus travels down the oviduct towards the uterus while continuing to divide mitotically without actually increasing in size, in a process called cleavage. After four divisions, the conceptus consists of 16 blastomeres, and it is known as the morula. Through the processes of compaction, cell division, and blastulation, the conceptus takes the form of the blastocyst by the fifth day of development, just as it approaches the site of implantation. When the blastocyst hatches from the zona pellucida, it can implant in the endometrial lining of the uterus and begin the embryonic stage of development. Figure 4-3 shows how a zygote continues to develop into an actual embryo. It shows that the endoderm of the embryo is then developed into internal organs, the mesoderm is developed into skeleton and muscles including heart, and ectoderm is developed into skin and nervous system.

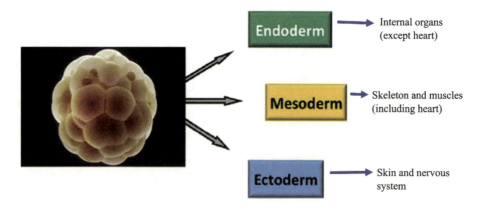

Figure 4-3　The Embryonic Stage of Development

NEUROLOGIC AND PSYCHOLOGIC DEVELOPMENT AFTER BIRTH

Table 4-1 lists the neurologic and psychologic development of the baby after birth.

Table 4-1　Neurologic and Psychologic Development After Birth

AGE	ACTIVITIES TO BE OBSERVED	ACTIVITIES RELATED BY PARENT
1-2 months	· Holds head erect and lifts head · Turns from side to back · Regards faces and follows objects through visual field · Drops toys · Becomes alert in response to voice	· Recognizes parent · Engages in vocalizations · Smiles spontaneously
3-5 months	· Grasps cube—first ulnar then later thumb opposition · Reaches for and brings objects to mouth · Makes "raspberry" sound · Sits with support	· Laughs · Anticipates food on sight · Turns from back to side
6-8 months	· Sits alone for a short period · Reaches with one hand · First scoops up a pellet then grasps it using thumb opposition · Imitates "bye-bye" · Passes object from hand to hand in midline · Babbles	· Rolls from back to stomach · Is inhibited by the word "no"
9-11 months	· Stands alone · Imitates pat-a-cack and peek-a-boo · Uses thumb and index finger to pick up pellet	· Walks by supporting self on furniture · Follows one-step verbal commands, eg, "Come here" "Give it to me"

AGE	ACTIVITIES TO BE OBSERVED	ACTIVITIES RELATED BY PARENT
1 year	· Walks independently · Says "mama" and "dada" with meaning · Can use a neat pincer grasp to pick up a pellet · Releases cube into cup after demonstration · Gives toys on request · Tries to build a tower of a 2 cubes	· Points to desired objects · Says 1 or 2 other words

A BRIEF INTRODUCTION OF COMMON HYPOEVOLUTISM HAPPENING DURING INFANCY

Growth retardation, mental retardation, language retardation, motor retardation, psychological retardation are the five clinical manifestations that could be recognized if hypoevolutism happens.

A variety of reasons could cause hypoevolutism.

① Normal growth and variation: this takes up to 80% - 90% of the total hypoevolutism, such as familial short stature, constitutional developmental delay and low birth weight caused short stature. These are related to congenital genetic factors or intrauterine dysplasia. The growth rate is basically normal and no special treatment is needed.

② Pathological causes: Such as chromosomal abnormalities (Down's syndrome, Turner syndrome), metabolic diseases, bone disease (osteochondral dysplasia), chronic diseases, chronic malnutrition, endocrine diseases such as growth hormone deficiency, etc, which causes hypothyroidism.

IN PERSON: A LATE DEVELOPER

This is a first person account of a mother talking about the late developments happening to her baby.

My son is 1 year and 8 months old. He started rolling only after 6 months and I thought he would sit by 8 – 10 months but he didn't do that. Instead, he used to roll back and forth even until he was 1 year old. I showed to a development specialist and they suggested for Physical Therapy. I started immediately and when he was 14 months he started to sit on his own and I continued the therapy and by 16 – 17 months he started crawling little and now he can crawl much better at 20 months. I had discontinued the therapy for about two months since he was 18 months. Now I started again with the therapy for him … He now is kneeling and holding furnitures with attempts to stand but he is scared to do that. When he tries to hold the walker to walk he cries and his right leg doesn't bend. He drags it instead and tries very rarely he lifts the legs. What could be the problem? The therapist says his legs are fine with length wise and not that stiff but slightly. I wonder what other problems could it be.

I would also like to clarify with this delayed milestones will this delay in his speech as well? Still doesn't say "mama" or "dada" when asked; he says his name not very clear though … and keeps telling only the word "aaahhh" most of the time. I wonder if my child will be alright, be like a normal child according to his age. Please advise.

Could you identify what the late developments of this child are according to the mother, and give her some suggestions on what she should do?

READING: BRIEFING THE WHOLE LIFE SPAN

The process begins with fertilization, where an egg released from the ovary of a female is penetrated by a sperm. The egg then lodges in the uterus, where an embryo and later a foetus develops until birth. Growth and development occur after birth, and include both physical and psychological development, influenced by genetic, hormonal, environmental and other factors. Development and growth continue throughout life, through childhood to puberty, and through adulthood to senility, and are referred to as the process of ageing.

The following part introduces puberty and adulthood for a little bit.

Puberty is the process of physical changes through which a child's body matures into an adult body capable of sexual reproduction. It is initiated by hormonal signals from the brain to the gonads: the ovaries in a girl, the testes in a boy. In response to the signals, the gonads produce hormones that stimulate libido and the growth, function, and transformation of the brain, bones, muscle, blood, skin, hair, breasts, and sex organs. Physical growth—height and weight—accelerates in the first half of puberty and is completed when an adult body has been developed. Until the maturation of their reproductive capabilities, the pre-pubertal physical differences between boys and girls are the external sex organs.

In human context, the term adult additionally has meanings associated with social and legal concepts. In contrast to a "minor", a legal adult is a person who has attained the age of majority and is therefore regarded as independent, self-sufficient, and responsible. Human adulthood encompasses psychological adult development. Definitions of adulthood are often inconsistent and contradictory; a person may be biologically an adult, and have adult behavior but still be treated as a child if they are under the legal age of majority. Conversely, one may legally be an adult but possess none of the maturity and responsibility that may define an adult.

Vocabulary

fertilization	/ˌfɜːtəlaɪˈzeɪʃn/	n.	受精,受精过程;受孕
infancy	/ˈɪnfənsi/	n.	婴儿期,幼儿期;初期
pediatrics	/ˌpiːdiˈætrɪks/	n.	小儿科;儿科学
heredity	/həˈredəti/	n.	遗传(过程);遗传特征
embryogenesis	/ˌembriəʊˈdʒenəsɪs/	n.	胚胎发生(形成),胚形成
foetus	/ˈfiːtəs/	n.	胎,胎儿
zygote	/ˈzaɪɡəʊt/	n.	[生物]合子,受精卵
synapsis	/sɪˈnæpsɪs/	n.	联会;突触;染色体结合
embryo	/ˈembriəʊ/	n.	胚,胚胎;(尤指受孕后八周内的)人类胚胎
conceptus	/kənˈseptəs/	n.	孕体
blastomere	/ˈblɑːstəmɪə/	n.	分裂球
endometrial	/ˌendʌˈmetrɪəl/	adj.	子宫内膜的
endoderm	/ˈendəʊdɜːm/	n.	内胚层
mesoderm	/ˈmesədɜːm/	n.	中胚层
ectoderm	/ˈektədɜːm/	n.	外胚层
retardation	/ˌriːtɑːˈdeɪʃn/	n.	延迟
hypoevolutism	/haɪpəʊevəˈluːtɪzəm/	n.	发育迟缓
manifestation	/ˌmænɪfeˈsteɪʃn/	n.	表示,显示
pathological	/ˌpæθəˈlɒdʒɪkl/	adj.	病理学的
Down's syndrome			唐氏综合征
Turner syndrome			特纳综合征
metabolic disease			代谢性疾病
osteochondral dysplasia			骨软骨发育不良
chronic disease			慢性病
endocrine disease			内分泌疾病

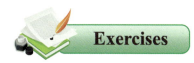

I *Try to define the following words and phrases in English.*

1. Fertilization: _____
2. Embryogenesis: _____
3. Clinical manifestation: _____
4. Osteochondral dysplasia: _____
5. Mental retardation: _____
6. Hypoevolutism: _____
7. Pathological cause: _____
8. Endoderm: _____
9. Endocrine disease: _____
10. Conceptus: _____

II *Match the listed words and phrases in the box with the definitions that follow.*

metabolic disease	endoderm	foetus
chronic disease	mesoderm	zygote
endocrine disease	ectoderm	embryo

1. A disease being long-lasting and recurrent or characterized by long suffering: _____
2. The outer germ layer that develops into skin and nervous tissue: _____
3. The cell resulting from the union of an ovum and a spermatozoon: _____

CHAPTER 5

MUSCULOSKELETAL SYSTEM
肌肉骨骼系统

Chapter Sections

Introduction

Bones

Vocabulary of bones

Joints

Vocabulary of joints

Muscles

Vocabulary of muscles

Terminology

Exercises

Chapter Goals

- To locate and name the major bones, joints, and muscles.
- To define terms relating to the structure and function of bones, joints, and muscles.
- To explain the motivation of joints.

INTRODUCTION

The **musculoskeletal system** includes the bones, muscles, and joints. All have important functions in the body.

Bones provide the framework on which the body is constructed and protect and support internal organs. Bones also assist the body in movement, because they serve as a point of attachment for muscles. Joints are the places at which bones come together. Several different types of joints are found within the body. The type of joint found in any specific location is determined by the need for greater or lesser flexibility of movement.

Muscles, whether attached to bones or to internal organs and blood vessels, are responsible for movement. Internal movement involves the contraction and relaxation of muscles found in viscera, and external movement is accomplished by the contraction and relaxation of muscles that are attached to the bones.

In this chapter, you will learn the names and features of the bones, muscles, and joints.

BONES

The precise number of bones in the adult human skeleton varies from one person to another, but on average there are 206 bones of varying shapes and sizes. The skeleton is divided into two main parts (Figure 5-1). The central bones of the skull, ribs, vertebral column (spine), and sternum (breastbone) form the **axial skeleton**. The bones of the arms and legs, along with the scapula (shoulder blade), clavicle (collar bone), and pelvis, make up the **appendicular skeleton.**

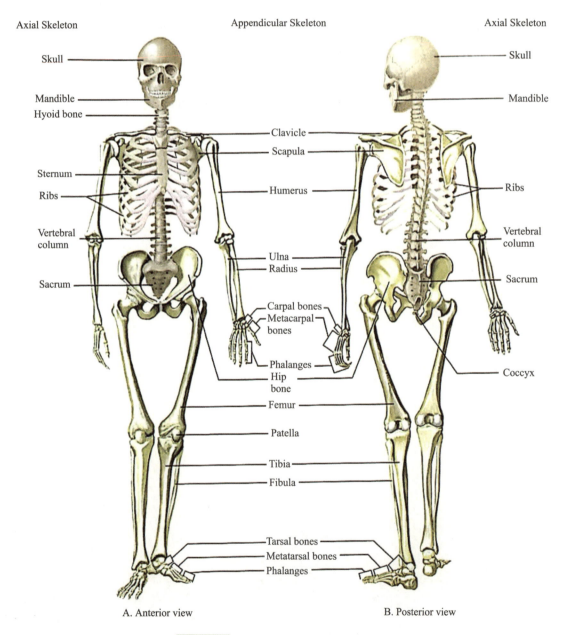

Figure 5-1　Divisions of the Skeletal System

Bone shapes

Bones are classified according to five main shapes (Figure 5-2):

Long bones are found in the thigh, lower leg, and upper and lower arm. These bones are very strong. They are broad at the ends where they join with other bones, and have large surface areas for muscle attachment.

Short bones are found in the wrist and ankle and are small with irregular shapes.

Flat bones are found covering soft body parts. These bones are the skull, shoulder blades, ribs and pelvic bones.

Irregular bones include vertebrae, the ilium (pelvis), and some skull bones, such as the sphenoid bone.

Sesamoid bones are small, rounded bones (resembling a sesame seed in shape). The patella is the largest example of a sesamoid bone.

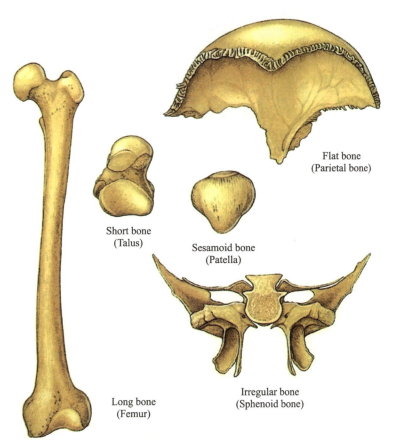

Figure 5-2 Bone Shapes

Bone Structure

The following is the anatomic divisions of a long bone such as the thigh bone or upper arm bone.

Figure 5-3 shows the regions of a long bone. The shaft, or middle region, of a long bone is called the **diaphysis.** Each end of a long bone is called the **epiphysis.**

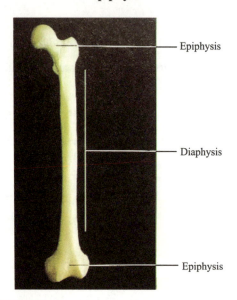

Figure 5-3　Regions of a Long Bone (anterior view)

Figure 5-4 shows the structure of a long bone.

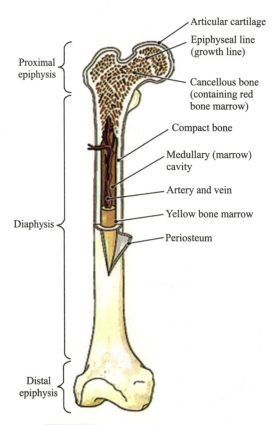

Figure 5-4　Structure of a Long Bone

The **periosteum** is a strong, fibrous, vascular membrane that covers the surface of long bones, except at the ends of the epiphyses. It has an extensive nerve supply as well. Bones other than long bones are also covered by the periosteum.

The ends of long bones and the surface of any bone that meets another bone to form a joint are covered with the **articular cartilage.** When two bones come together to form a joint, the bones themselves do not touch precisely. The articular cartilage that caps the end of one bone comes into contact with that of the other bone. Articular cartilage is a very smooth, strong, and slick tissue. It cushions the joint and allows it to move smoothly and efficiently.

The compact (cortical) bone is a layer of hard, dense bone that lies under the periosteum in all bones and is located chiefly around the diaphysis of long bones. The compact bone is tunneled out in the central shaft of the long bones by a **medullary cavity** that contains **yellow bone marrow**, arteries and veins.

The cancellous bone, sometimes called **the spongy bone**, is much more porous and less dense than compact bone. Spaces in cancellous bone contain **red bone marrow**. The red bone marrow consists of immature and mature blood cells in various stages of development. **Hematopoiesis** (poiesis means formation) is the production of all types of blood cells in the bone marrow.

Cranial Bones

The bones of the skull, or cranium, protect the brain and structures related to it, such as the sense organs. Muscles for controlling head movements and chewing motions are connected to the cranial bones (Figure 5-5). The cranial bones join each other at joints called **sutures**.

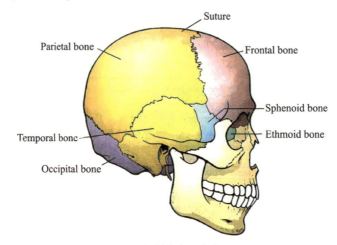

A. Right lateral view

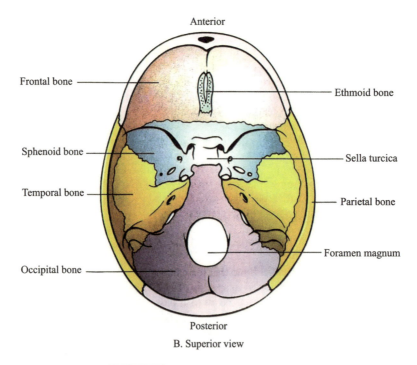

B. Superior view

Figure 5-5　Regions of Cranial Bones

Vertebral Column

The **vertebral (spinal) column** is composed of 26 bone segments, called **vertebrae**, which are arranged in five divisions from the base of the skull to the tailbone. The divisions of the vertebral column is: **cervical vertebrae**, **thoracic vertebrae**, **lumbar vertebrae**, **sacrum**, and **coccyx** (Figure 5-6).

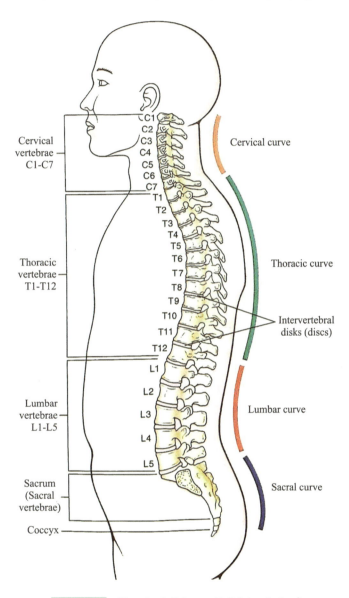

Figure 5-6 Vertebral Column (left lateral view)

When viewed from the side with the subject facing to the left, the vertebral column shows four curves (cervical, thoracic, lumbar, sacral), two of which are convex and two of which are concave. The curves of the column, like the curves in a long bone, are important because they increase its strength, help maintain balance in the upright position, absorb shocks from walking, and help protect the column from fracture.

Although the individual vertebrae in the separate regions of the spinal column are all slightly different in structure, they do have several parts in common.

A vertebra (Figure 5-7) is composed of an inner, thick, the round anterior portion called the **vertebral body**. Between the body of one vertebra and the body of another vertebra lying beneath or above is an **intervertebral disk (disc)**. This is a pad of cartilage that provides flexibility and absorbs shocks to the vertebral column.

The posterior portion of a vertebra (**vertebral arch**) consists of a single **spinous process**, a **transverse process**, one on each side of the spinous process, and a bar-like **lamina** between each transverse process and the spinous process. The neural or **spinal canal** is the space between the vertebral body and the vertebral arch through which the spinal cord passes.

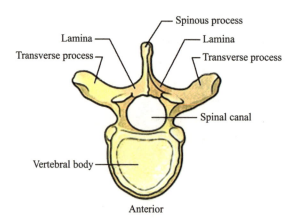

Figure 5-7　Typical Vertebra (superior view)

CHAPTER 5 MUSCULOSKELETAL SYSTEM 49

 Example Bones of the Thorax, Pelvis and Extremities

Figures 5-8, 5-9, 5-10 and 5-11 show example bones of the thorax, pelvis and extremities.

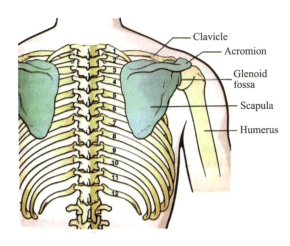

Figure 5-8 Thorax

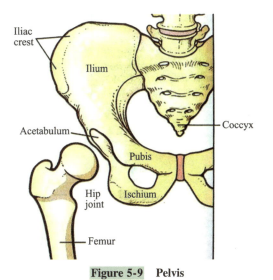

Figure 5-9 Pelvis

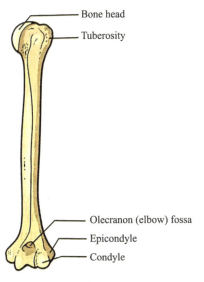

Figure 5-10 Upper Extremity (Humerus, upper arm bone)

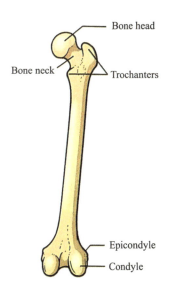

Figure 5-11 Lower Extremity (Femur, thigh bone)

Vocabulary of Bones

skeleton	/ˈskelɪtn/	n.	骨骼,骨架
musculoskeletal	/ˌmʌskjələʊˈskelətəl/	adj.	肌(与)骨骼的
axial skeleton	/ˈæksɪəl/		中轴骨
appendicular skeleton	/ˌæpənˈdɪkjələ/		四肢骨骼,附肢骨骼
irregular bone	/ɪˈreɡjələ/		不规则骨
sesamoid bone	/ˈsesəmɔɪd/		籽骨
diaphysis	/daɪˈæfəsɪs/	n.	骨干
epiphysis	/ɪˈpɪfɪsɪs; e-/	n.	骨骺
periosteum	/ˌperɪˈɒstɪəm/	n.	骨膜
cartilage	/ˈkɑːrtɪlɪdʒ/	n.	软骨
compact (cortical) bone	/ˈkɒmpækt ˈkɔːtɪkəl/		密质骨;骨密质;致密骨
cancellous bone	/ˈkænsələs/		松质骨
red bone marrow	/ˈmærəʊ/		红骨髓
hematopoiesis	/ˌhemətəʊpɔɪˈisɪs/	n.	造血作用
cranial bone	/ˈkreɪnɪəl/		颅骨,头骨
vertebra	/ˈvɜːtɪbrə/	n.	椎骨
cervical	/ˈsɜːvɪkl/	adj.	颈的
thoracic	/θɔːˈræsɪk/	adj.	胸的;胸廓的
lumbar	/ˈlʌmbə/	n. adj.	腰椎 腰的;腰部的
sacrum	/ˈseɪkrəm/	n.	骶骨
disk (disc)	/dɪsk/	n.	椎间盘
spinal canal	/ˈspaɪnl kəˈnæl/		椎管
acromion	/əˈkrəʊmɪən/	n.	肩峰
malleolus	/məˈlɪələs/	n.	踝
olecranon	/əʊˈlekrənɒn/	n.	鹰嘴(肘部的骨性隆起);肘突
suture	/ˈsuːtʃə(r)/	n.	纤维性关节
acetabulum	/æsəˈtæbjʊləm/	n.	髋臼;关节窝

JOINTS

The study of the joints between bones is called **arthrology**. The joints themselves are known as **articulations. Joints** are important because they are the points of movement of the body. They can suffer significant trauma or diseases. Diseases such as arthritis affect millions of people worldwide.

Types of Joints

A joint (articulation) is a coming together of two or more bones. The three major groups of joints classified according to their composition are fibrous, cartilaginous, and synovial joints.

Fibrous joints (Figure 5-12) are composed of connective tissue fibers between two bones. They permit little movement.

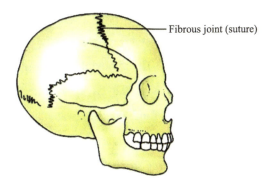

Figure 5-12 Fibrous Joint

Cartilaginous joints (Figure 5-13) consist of cartilage between two bones and are generally more movable than fibrous joints, although some cartilaginous joints may have no movement at all.

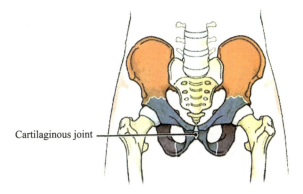

Figure 5-13 Cartilaginous Joint

Synovial joints (Figure 5-14) have the most complex structure, including a **joint (articular) capsule**, an inner membrane, and synovial fluid, and they are the most movable of the joints.

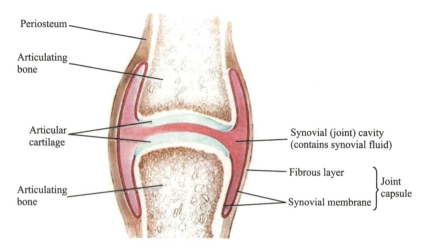

Figure 5-14　Synovial Joint

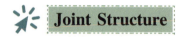 Joint Structure

The bones in a synovial joint(Figure 5-15) are surrounded by a **joint capsule** composed of fibrous tissue. Ligaments (thickened fibrous bands of connective tissue) anchor one bone to another and thereby add considerable strength to the joint capsule in critical areas. Bones at the joint are covered with a smooth, glistening white tissue called the **articular cartilage**. The **synovial membrane** lies under the joint capsule and lines the **synovial cavity** between the bones. The synovial cavity is filled with a special lubricating fluid produced by the synovial membrane. This **synovial fluid** contains water and nutrients that nourish as well as lubricate the joints so that friction on the articular cartilage is minimal.

A **meniscus** is a crescent-shaped fibrocartilaginous structure that partly divides a joint cavity and acts as a protective cushion. It is present in the knee.

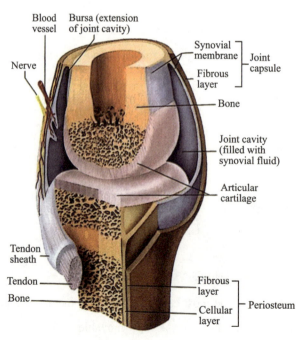

Figure 5-15　Synovial Joint Structure

Motivation of Synovial Joints

In a synovial joint, the shape of articular cartilage surfaces and the way they fit together determine the range and direction of the joints movement (Figure 5-16).

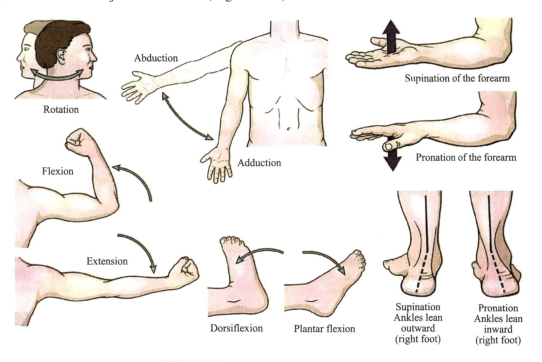

Figure 5-16　Motivation of Synovial Joints

Vocabulary of Joints

arthrology	/ɑːˈθrɒlədʒi/	n.	关节学
articulation	/ɑːˌtɪkjuˈleɪʃn/	n.	关节;关节连接
synovial joint	/sɪˈnəʊviəl, saɪ-/	n.	滑液关节;滑膜关节
ligament	/ˈlɪgəmənt/	n.	韧带
meniscus	/məˈnɪskəs/	n.	半月板
synovial membrane	/sɪˈnəʊviəl ˈmembreɪn/	n.	滑膜;滑液膜
synovial cavity	/sɪˈnəʊviəl ˈkævəti/		滑膜腔
synovial fluid	/sɪˈnəʊviəl ˈfluːɪd/		滑液
flexion	/ˈflekʃn/	n.	弯曲,屈曲
extension	/ɪkˈstenʃn/	n.	伸展

abduction	/æbˈdʌkʃn/	n.	外展
adduction	/əˈdʌkʃn/	n.	内收
rotation	/rəʊˈteɪʃn/	n.	旋转
dorsiflexion	/ˌdɔːsiˈflekʃn/	n.	背屈
plantar flexion	/ˈplæntə/		跖屈
supination	/ˌsuːpəˈneɪʃn/	n.	旋后
pronation	/prəʊˈneɪʃn/	n.	旋前

MUSCLES

There are three types of muscle tissue in the human body: smooth muscle, cardiac muscle, and skeletal muscle, also known as myocardium (Figure 5-17).

The smooth muscle, which is found in the walls of internal organs such as the intestines, is made of short spindle-shaped fibers packed together in layers.

The cardiac muscle, found only in heart, has short, interconnecting fibers.

The skeletal muscle is composed of bundles of long, striated fibers (cells).

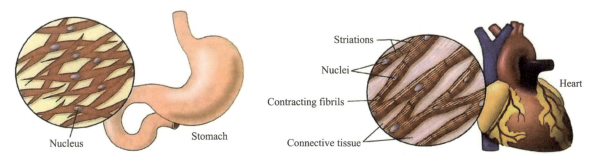

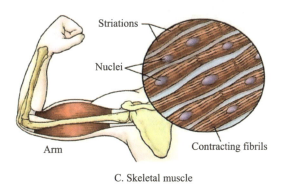

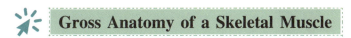

Figure 5-17 Types of Muscles

Gross Anatomy of a Skeletal Muscle

There are over 600 skeletal muscles (Figure 5-18 and Figure 5-19) in the human body. The skeletal muscles make up nearly half the total weight of the human body and provide the forces that enable the body to move and maintain its posture.

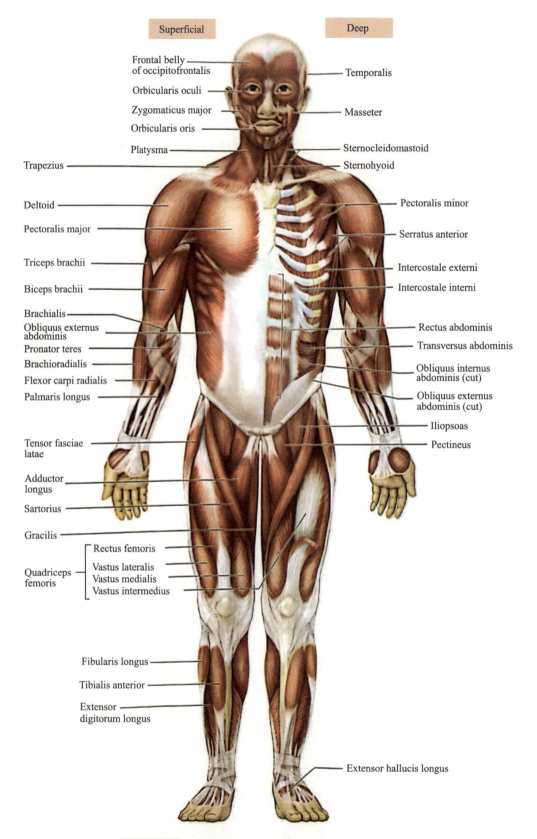

Figure 5-18 Divisions of Skeletal Muscles (anterior view)

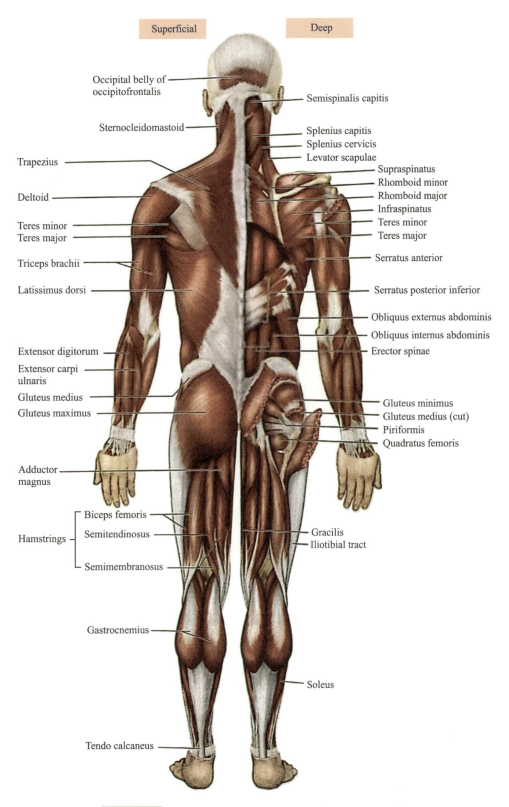

Figure 5-19 Divisions of Skeletal Muscles (posterior view)

Origin and Insertion

Skeletal muscles produce movements by exerting force on **tendons**, which in turn pull on bones. Ordinarily, the attachment of a muscle tendon to the stationary bone is called the **origin**. The attachment of the other muscle tendon to the movable bone is the **insertion**. A good analogy is a spring on a door. The part of the spring attached to the door represents the insertion; the part attached to the frame is the origin. The fleshy portion of the muscle between the tendons of the origin and insertion is called the **belly** (Figure 5-20).

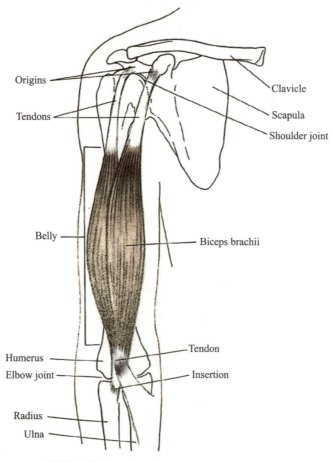

Figure 5-20 Origin and Insertion of the Muscle

Group Actions in Skeletal Muscle

Most movements are coordinated by several skeletal muscles acting in groups rather than individually and most skeletal muscles are arranged in opposing pairs at joints, that is, flexors-extensors, abductors-adductors, and so on. Consider flexing the forearm at the elbow, for example. A muscle that causes a desired action is referred to as the prime mover (**agonist**). In this instance, the biceps brachii is the **prime mover**. Simultaneously with the contraction of the biceps brachii, another muscle, called the **antagonist**, is relaxing. In this movement, the triceps brachii serves as the antagonist. The antagonist has an effect opposite to that of the prime mover, that is, the antagonist relaxes and yields to the movement of the prime mover(Figure 5-21).

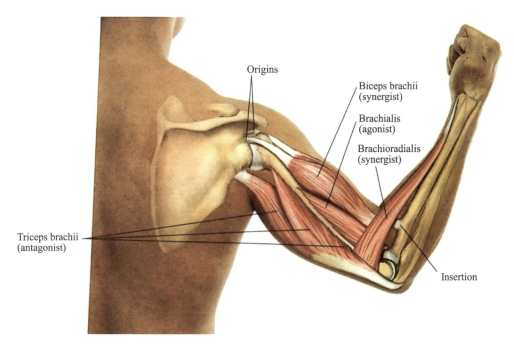

Figure 5-21 Agonist and Antagonist

Types of Muscular Actions

Not all muscle contractions produce movement. In an **isometric contraction**, there is a minimal shortening of the muscle. It remains nearly the same length, but the tension on the muscle increases greatly. Although isometric contractions do not result in body movement, energy is still expended. You can demonstrate such a contraction by carrying your books with your arm extended. The weight of the books pulls the arm downward, stretching the shoulder and arm muscles.

A contraction that does produce movement is an **isotonic contraction** (iso = equal; tonos = tension). Isotonic contractions are probably familiar to you. As the contraction occurs, the muscle shortens and pulls on another structure, such as a bone, to produce movement. During such a contraction, the tension remains constant and energy is expended.

Vocabulary of Muscles

cardiac	/ˈkɑːdiæk/	adj.	心脏的；心脏病的
myocardium	/ˌmaɪəˈkɑːdɪəm/	n.	心肌
skeletal muscle	/ˈskelətl/		骨骼肌
tendon	/ˈtendən/	n.	腱
insertion	/ɪnˈsɜːʃn/	n.	插入；插入点
agonist	/ˈæɡənɪst/	n.	主动肌
antagonist	/ænˈtæɡənɪst/	n.	拮抗肌
isometric contraction	/ˌaɪsəˈmetrɪk/		等长收缩
isotonic contraction	/ˌaɪsəˈtɒnɪk/		等张收缩
trapezius	/trəˈpiːzjəs/	n.	斜方肌
deltoid	/ˈdeltɔɪd/	n.	三角肌
pectoralis major	/ˈpektərəlɪs/		胸大肌
biceps brachii	/ˈbaɪseps ˈbreɪkɪaɪ/		肱二头肌
brachial	/ˈbreɪkɪəl/	adj.	臂的
hamstring	/ˈhæmstrɪŋ/	n.	腘绳肌
quadriceps femoris	/ˈkwɒdrɪseps feˈməʊrɪz/		股四头肌

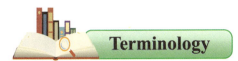

BONES AND MUSCLES

frontal bone	/ˈfrʌntl bəʊn/	额骨
parietal bone	/pəˈraɪətəl bəʊn/	顶骨
temporal bone	/ˈtempərəl bəʊn/	颞骨
occipital bone	/ɒkˈsɪpətəl bəʊn/	枕骨
sphenoid bone	/ˈsfiːnɔɪd bəʊn/	蝶骨
ethmoid bone	/eθˈmɔɪd bəʊn/	筛骨
scapula	/ˈskæpjələ/	肩胛骨
clavicle	/ˈklævɪkl/	锁骨
manubrium sterni	/məˈnjuːbrɪəm/	胸骨柄
body of sternum	/ˈstɜːrnəm/	胸骨体
xiphoid process	/ˈzɪfɔɪd ˈprəʊses/	剑突
rib	/rɪb/	肋骨
cervical vertebrae	/ˈsɜːrvɪkl ˈvɜːtɪbreɪ/	颈椎
thoracic vertebrae	/θɔːˈræsɪk ˈvɜːtɪbreɪ/	胸椎
lumbar vertebrae	/ˈlʌmbə(r) ˈvɜːtɪbreɪ/	腰椎
humerus	/ˈhjuːmərəs/	肱骨
radius	/ˈreɪdiəs/	桡骨
ulna	/ˈʌlnə/	尺骨
carpal bone	/ˈkɑːrpl bəʊn/	腕骨
metacarpal bone	/ˌmetəˈkɑːrpl bəʊn/	掌骨
phalange	/ˈfælændʒ/	指骨
scaphoid bone	/ˈskæfɔɪd bəʊn/	手舟骨
lunate bone	/ˈluːneɪt bəʊn/	月骨
triquetral bone	/traɪˈkwetr(ə)l bəʊn/	三角骨
pisiform bone	/ˈpɪzɪfɔːm bəʊn/	豌豆骨
trapezium bone	/trəˈpiːziəm bəʊn/	大多角骨
trapezoid bone	/ˈtræpəˌzɔɪd bəʊn/	小多角骨
capitate bone	/ˈkæpəteɪt bəʊn/	头状骨
hamate bone	/ˈheɪmeɪt bəʊn/	钩骨

pelvis	/ˈpelvɪs/	骨盆
sacrum	/ˈseɪkrəm, ˈsæ-/	骶骨
coccyx	/ˈkɒksɪks/	尾骨
hip bone	/hɪp bəʊn/	髋骨
ilium	/ˈɪliəm/	髂骨
ischium	/ˈɪskiəm/	坐骨
pubis	/ˈpjuːbɪs/	耻骨
femur	/ˈfiːmə(r)/	股骨
patella	/pəˈtelə/	髌骨
tibia	/ˈtɪbiə/	胫骨
fibula	/ˈfɪbjələ/	腓骨
tarsal bone	/ˈtɑːsl bəʊn/	跗骨
talus	/ˈteɪləs/	距骨
calcaneus	/kælˈkeɪniəs/	跟骨
navicular bone	/nəˈvɪkjʊlə(r) bəʊn/	足舟骨
medial cuneiform bone	/ˈmiːdiəl ˈkjuːnɪfɔːm bəʊn/	内侧楔骨
intermedius cuneiform bone	/ɪntəˈmiːdiəs ˈkjuːnɪfɔːm bəʊn/	中间楔骨
lateral cuneiform bone	/ˈlætərəl ˈkjuːnɪfɔːm bəʊn/	外侧楔骨
cuboid bone	/ˈkjuːbɔɪd bəʊn/	骰骨
metatarsal bone	/ˌmetəˈtɑːsl bəʊn/	跖骨
phalange	/ˈfælændʒ/	趾骨
occipitofrontalis	/ɒksɪpɪtɔːfrʌntˈlɪs/	枕额肌
orbicularis oculi	/ɔːˌbɪkjʊˈlɑːrɪs ˈɒkjʊli/	眼轮匝肌
zygomaticus major	/zaɪɡəˈmætɪkəs ˈmeɪdʒə(r)/	颧大肌
orbicularis oris	/ɔːˌbɪkjʊˈlɑːrɪs ˈɒrɪs/	口轮匝肌
platysma	/pləˈtɪzmə/	颈阔肌
temporalis	/ˌtempəˈreɪlɪs/	颞肌
masseter	/mæˈseɪtə/	咬肌
sternocleidomastoid	/ˌstɜːnə(ʊ)ˌklaɪdə(ʊ)ˈmæstɔɪd/	胸锁乳突肌
sternohyoid	/ˌstɜːnəʊˈhaɪɔɪd/	胸骨舌骨肌
semispinalis capitis	/ˌsemɪspaɪˈnælɪs ˈkæpɪtɪs/	头半棘肌
semispinalis cervicis	/ˌsemɪspaɪˈnælɪs ˈsɜːvɪsɪs/	颈半棘肌
scalene	/ˈskeɪliːn/	斜角肌
levator scapulae	/lɪˈveɪtə(r) ˈskæpjʊliː/	肩胛提肌

trapezius	/trəˈpiːziəs/	斜方肌
deltoid	/ˈdeltɔɪd/	三角肌
pectoralis major	/ˈpektərəlɪs ˈmeɪdʒə(r)/	胸大肌
pectoralis minor	/ˈpektərəlɪs ˈmaɪnə(r)/	胸小肌
biceps brachii	/ˈbaɪseps ˈbreɪkɪaɪ/	肱二头肌
triceps brachii	/ˈtraɪseps ˈbreɪkɪaɪ/	肱三头肌
brachialis	/ˈbreɪkjəlɪs/	肱肌
brachioradialis	/breɪtʃiəˈreɪdiəlɪs/	肱桡肌
latissimus dorsi	/leɪˈtɪsɪməs ˈdɔːsi/	背阔肌
rhomboid major	/ˈrɒmbɔɪd ˈmeɪdʒə(r)/	大菱形肌
rhomboid minor	/ˈrɒmbɔɪd ˈmaɪnə(r)/	小菱形肌
serratus anterior	/seˈreɪtəs ænˈtɪəriə(r)/	前锯肌
serratus posterior inferior	/seˈreɪtəs pɒˈstɪəriə(r) ɪnˈfɪəriə(r)/	下后锯肌
subclavius	/sʌbˈklæviəs/	锁骨下肌
coracobrachialis	/kɒrəkəʊbˈrækjəlɪs/	喙肱肌
teres major	/ˈteriːz ˈmeɪdʒə(r)/	大圆肌
supraspinatus	/sʌprɑːspɪˈneɪtəs/	冈上肌
teres minor	/ˈteriːz ˈmaɪnə(r)/	小圆肌
infraspinatus	/iːnfrəspɪˈneɪtəs/	冈下肌
subscapularis	/sʌbˈskæpjʊˈleərɪs/	肩胛下肌
anconeus	/æŋˈkəʊniəs/	肘肌
supinator	/ˈsjuːpɪneɪtə/	旋后肌
pronator teres	/prəʊˈneɪtə(r) ˈteriːz/	旋前圆肌
intercostale externi	/ˌɪntəˈkɒstl ɪkˈstɜːrnɪ/	肋间外肌
intercostale interni	/ˌɪntəˈkɒstl ɪnˈtɜːrni/	肋间内肌
rectus abdominis	/ˈrektəs æbˈdɒmɪnɪs/	腹直肌
transversus abdominis	/trænzˈvɜːsəs æbˈdɒmɪnɪs/	腹横肌
obliquus externus abdominis	/əˈbliːkwəs eksˈtɜːrnəs æbˈdɒmɪnɪs/	腹外斜肌
obliquus internus abdominis	/əˈbliːkwəs ɪnˈtɜːrnəs æbˈdɒmɪnɪs/	腹内斜肌
erector spinae	/ɪˈrektə ˈspaɪniː/	竖脊肌
flexor carpi radialis	/ˈfleksə(r) ˈkɑːpaɪ reɪdɪˈeɪlɪs/	桡侧腕屈肌
flexor carpi ulnaris	/ˈfleksə(r) ˈkɑːpaɪ ˈʌlnərɪz/	尺侧腕屈肌
pronator quadratus	/prəʊˈneɪtə kwɒˈdreɪtəs/	旋前方肌
palmar interossei	/ˈpælmə ɪntɜːrɒˈziː/	掌侧骨间肌

palmaris longus	/ˈpælmrɪs ˈlɒŋɡʌs/	掌长肌
extensor digitorum	/ɪksˈtensər ˈdɪdʒɪˈtɒrəm/	指伸肌
extensor carpi radialis brevis	/ɪksˈtensər ˈkɑːpaɪ reɪdɪˈeɪlɪs brevɪs/	桡侧腕短伸肌
extensor carpi radialis longus	/ɪksˈtensər ˈkɑːpaɪ reɪdɪˈeɪlɪs ˈlɒŋɡʌs/	桡侧腕长伸肌
extensor carpi ulnaris	/ɪkˈstensər ˈkɑːpaɪ ˈʌlnərɪz/	尺侧腕伸肌
gluteus maximus	/ˈɡluːtiəs ˈmæksɪməs/	臀大肌
gluteus medius	/ˈɡluːtiəs ˈmiːdɪəs/	臀中肌
gluteus minimus	/ˈɡluːtiəs ˈmɪnɪməs/	臀小肌
iliopsoas	/ɪliəʊˈsəʊəs/	髂腰肌
pectineus	/pekˈtɪnɪəs/	耻骨肌
piriformis	/ˌpɪrəˈfɔːmɪs/	梨状肌
quadratus femoris	/kwɒˈdreɪtəs feˈməʊrɪz/	股方肌
quadratus lumborum	/kwɒˈdreɪtəs ləmˈbɔːrəm/	腰方肌
tensor fasciae latae	/ˈtensə(r) ˈfæʃɪɪ ˈleɪtiː/	阔筋膜张肌
adductor longus	/əˈdʌktə(r) ˈlɒŋɡʌs/	长收肌
adductor magnus	/əˈdʌktə(r) ˈmæɡnəs/	大收肌
adductor brevis	/əˈdʌktə(r) brevɪs/	短收肌
quadriceps femoris	/ˈkwɒdrɪseps feˈməʊrɪz/	股四头肌
rectus femoris	/ˈrektəs feˈməʊrɪz/	股直肌
vastus medialis	/ˈvɑːstəs ˈmiːdɪɑːlɪs/	股内侧肌
vastus intermedius	/ˈvɑːstəs ɪntərˈmiːdɪəs/	股中间肌
vastus lateralis	/ˈvɑːstəs ˈlætərɑːlɪs/	股外侧肌
biceps femoris	/ˈbaɪseps feˈməʊrɪz/	股二头肌
sartorius	/sɑːˈtɔːrɪəs/	缝匠肌
semitendinosus	/ˌsemɪˌtendɪˈnəʊsəs/	半腱肌
semimembranosus	/ˌsemɪˌmembrəˈnəʊsəs/	半膜肌
gracilis	/ˈɡræsɪlɪs/	股薄肌
popliteus	/pɒpˈlɪtɪəs/	腘肌
iliotibial tract	/ɪliəʊˈtɪbɪəl trækt/	髂胫束
gastrocnemius	/ˌɡæstrɒkˈniːmɪəs/	腓肠肌
soleus	/ˈsɒlɪəs/	比目鱼肌
fibularis longus	/ˌfɪbjʊˈlærɪs ˈlɒŋɡʌs/	腓骨长肌
flexor digitorum brevis	/ˈfleksə(r) dɪdʒɪˈtɒrʌm brevɪs/	趾短屈肌
flexor digitorum longus	/ˈfleksə(r) dɪdʒɪˈtɒrʌm ˈlɒŋɡʌs/	趾长屈肌

tibialis anterior	/ˈtɪbɪəlɪs ænˈtɪərɪə(r)/	胫骨前肌
tibialis posterior	/ˈtɪbɪəlɪs pɒˈstɪərɪə(r)/	胫骨后肌
extensor digitorum brevis	/ɪksˈtensər ˈdɪdʒɪˈtɒrʌm brevɪs/	趾短伸肌
extensor digitorum longus	/ɪksˈtensər ˈdɪdʒɪˈtɒrʌm ˈlɒŋgʌs/	趾长伸肌
tendon calcaneus	/ˈtendən kælˈkeɪnɪəs/	跟腱

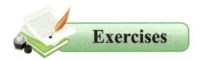

Exercises

I *Match the name with each numbered part and write the number in the corresponding blank.*

1. THE SKELETON

_____ Radius   _____ Facial bones
_____ Vertebral column   _____ Mandible
_____ Humerus   _____ Sternum
_____ Ribs   _____ Tarsal bones
_____ Scapula   _____ Sacrum
_____ Cranium   _____ Calcaneus
_____ Carpals   _____ Metacarpals
_____ Fibula   _____ Pelvis
_____ Ilium   _____ Femur
_____ Patella   _____ Phalanges
_____ Metatarsals   _____ Clavicle
_____ Ulna   _____ Tibia

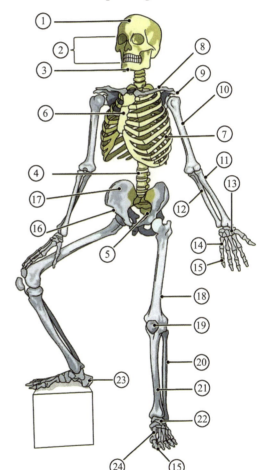

2. VERTEBRAL COLUMN

_____ Body of vertebra

_____ Coccyx

_____ Sacrum

_____ Lumbar vertebrae

_____ Thoracic vertebrae

_____ Intervertebral disk

_____ Cervical vertebrae

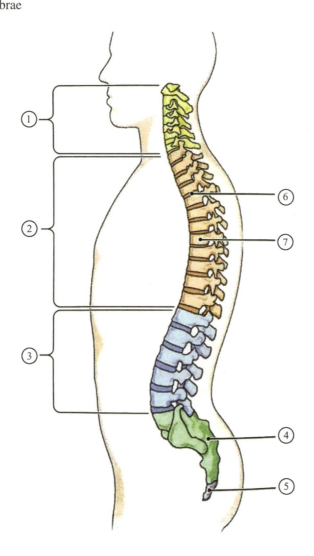

3. SUPERFICIAL MUSCLES, ANTERIOR VIEW

_____ Intercostale interni

_____ Serratus anterior

_____ Trapezius

_____ Masseter

_____ Triceps brachii

_____ Orbicularis oris

_____ Extensor carpi

_____ Pectoralis major

_____ Adductors of thigh

_____ Sternocleidomastoid

_____ Biceps brachii

_____ Temporalis

_____ Flexor carpi radialis

_____ Deltoid

_____ Obliquus externus abdominis

_____ Fibularis longus

_____ Rectus abdominis

_____ Brachioradialis

_____ Tibialis anterior

_____ Orbicularis oculi

_____ Quadriceps femoris

_____ Gastrocnemius

_____ Soleus

_____ Obliquus internus abdominis

_____ Sartorius

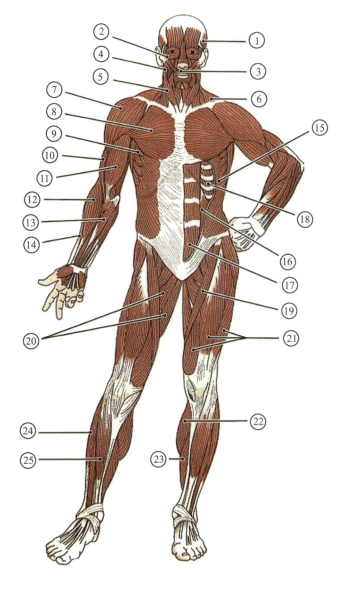

4. SUPERFICIAL MUSCLES, POSTERIOR VIEW

_____ Latissimus dorsi
_____ Triceps brachii
_____ Gluteus maximus
_____ Gluteus medius
_____ Teres major
_____ Sternocleidomastoid
_____ Fibularis longus
_____ Teres minor
_____ Deltoid
_____ Gastrocnemius
_____ Hamstring group
_____ Trapezius

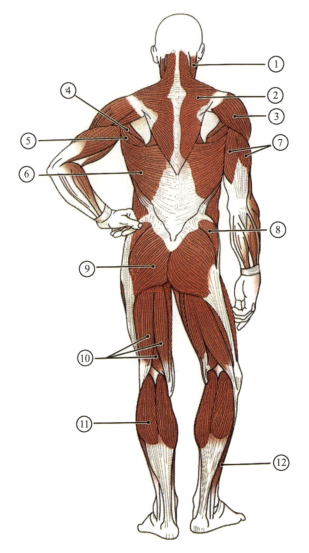

Ⅱ *Reading comprehension.*

The Superficial Back Muscles

The muscles of the back can be divided into three groups—superficial, intermediate and deep.

Superficial—associated with movements of the shoulder.

Intermediate—associated with movements of the thoracic cage.

Deep—associated with movements of the vertebral column.

The deep muscles develop embryologically in the back, and are thus described as intrinsic muscles. The superficial and intermediate muscles do not develop in the back, and are classified as extrinsic muscles.

This article is about the anatomy of the superficial back muscles—their attachments, innervations and functions.

The superficial back muscles (Figure 5-22) are situated underneath the skin and superficial fascia. They originate from the vertebral column and attach to the bones of the shoulder—the clavicle, scapula and humerus. All these muscles are therefore associated with movements of the upper limb.

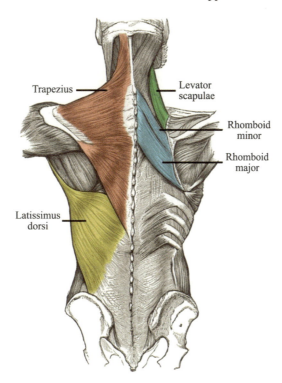

Figure 5-22 The Superficial Muscles of the Back

The muscles in this group are the trapezius, latissimus dorsi, levator scapulae and the rhomboids. The trapezius and the latissimus dorsi lie the most superficially, with the trapezius covering the rhomboids and levator scapulae.

(1) Trapezius

The trapezius is a broad, flat and triangular muscle. The muscles on each side form a trapezoid shape. It is the most superficial of all the back muscles.

Attachments: The trapezius originates from the skull, ligamentum nuchae and the spinous processes of C7-T12. The fibres attach to the clavicle, acromion and the scapula spine.

Innervation: Motor innervation is from the accessory nerve. It also receives proprioceptor fibres from C3 and C4 spinal nerves.

Actions: The upper fibres of the trapezius elevate the scapula and rotate it during abduction of the arm. The middle fibres retract the scapula and the lower fibres pull the scapula inferiorly.

(2) Latissimus Dorsi

The latissimus dorsi originates from the lower part of the back, where it covers a wide area.

Attachments: The latissimus dorsi has a broad origin—arising from the spinous processes of T6-T12, iliac crest, thoracolumbar fascia and the inferior three ribs. The fibres converge into a tendon that attaches to the intertubercular sulcus of the humerus.

Innervation: Thoracodorsal nerve.

Actions: It extends, adducts and medially rotates the upper limb.

(3) Levator Scapulae

The levator scapulae is a small strap-like muscle. It begins in the neck, and descends to attach to the scapula.

Attachments: The levator scapulae originates from the transverse processes of the C1-C4 vertebrae and attaches to the medial border of the scapula.

Innervation: Dorsal scapular nerve.

Actions: It elevates the scapula.

(4) Rhomboids

There are two rhomboid muscles—rhomboid major and rhomboid minor. The rhomboid minor is situated superiorly to the rhomboid major.

(5) Rhomboid Major

Attachments: The rhomboid major originates from the spinous processes of T1-T4 vertebrae. It attaches to the medial border of the scapula, between the scapula spine and inferior angle.

Innervation: Dorsal scapular nerve.

Actions: It retracts and rotates the scapula.

(6) Rhomboid Minor

Attachments: The rhomboid minor originates from the spinous processes of C6-C7 vertebrae. It attaches to the medial border of the scapula, at the level of the spine of scapula.

Innervation: Dorsal scapular nerve.

Actions: It retracts and rotates the scapula.

(　　) 1. Which superficial muscle of the back is most important in allowing a shrugging motion?

  A. Trapezius.   B. Rhomboid major.

  C. Rhomboid minor.   D. Levator scapulae.

(　　) 2. Which muscle attaches specifically to the spinous processes of the T1-T4 vertebrae?

  A. Rhomboid major.   B. Rhomboid minor.

    C. Trapezius.   D. Levator scapulae.

(   ) 3. Which of these nerves innervates latissimus dorsi?

    A. Glossopharyngeal nerve.   B. Dorsal scapular nerve.

    C. Long thoracic nerve.   D. Thoracodorsal nerve.

CHAPTER 6

NERVOUS SYSTEM
神经系统

Chapter Sections

Introduction

The neuron

Nerves

The brain

Protecting the brain

The spinal cord

The spinal nerves

Reflexes

The autonomic nervous system

Vocabulary

Exercises

Chapter Goals

- To name and locate the nervous system.
- To describe the components of the nervous system.
- To describe the regions of the brain and their functions.

INTRODUCTION

The nervous system and the endocrine system coordinate and control the body. Together they regulate our responses to the environment and maintain homeostasis. Whereas the endocrine system functions by means of circulating hormones, the nervous system functions by means of electric impulses and locally released chemicals called neurotransmitters. For study purposes, the nervous system may be divided structurally into two parts (Figure 6-1).

(1) The **central nervous system** (**CNS**), consisting of the brain and spinal cord.

(2) The **peripheral nervous system** (**PNS**), consisting of all nervous tissue outside the brain and spinal cord.

Functionally, the nervous system can be divided into two systems.

(1) **The somatic nervous system**, which controls skeletal muscles.

(2) **The visceral** or **autonomic nervous system** (**ANS**), which controls smooth muscle, cardiac muscle, and glands. The ANS regulates responses to stress and helps maintain homeostasis.

Two types of cells are found in the nervous system. **Neurons**, or nerve cells, make up the conducting tissue of the nervous system. **Neuroglia** are the cells that support and protect nervous tissue.

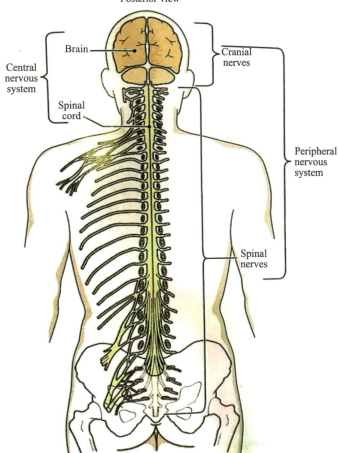

Figure 6-1 Anatomic Divisions of the Nervous System

THE NEURON

The neuron is the nervous system's basic functional unit. It is a microscopic structure. Impulses pass along the parts of a nerve cell in a definite manner and direction. The parts of a neuron are pictured in Figure 6-2.

(1) **Dendrites**: A stimulus begins an impulse in the branching fibers of the neuron.

(2) **Cell body**: A change in the electrical charge of the dendrite membranes is thus begin, and the nervous impulse moves along the dendrites like the movement of falling dominoes. The impulse, traveling in only one direction, next reaches the cell body.

(3) **Cell nucleus**: Which is in the cell body.

(4) **Axon**: Extending from the cell body is the axon, which carries the impulse away from the cell body. Axons can be covered with a fatty tissue called myelin.

(5) **Myelin sheath**: The purpose of this myelin sheath is to insulate the axon and speed transmission of the electrical impulse. The myelin sheath gives a white appearance to the nerve fiber—hence the term white matter, as in parts of the spinal cord and the white matter of the brain and most peripheral nerves. The gray matter of the brain and spinal cord is composed of the cell bodies of neurons that appear gray because they are not covered by a myelin sheath.

(6) **Terminal end fibers**: The nervous impulse passes through the axon to leave the cell via the terminal end fibers of the neuron.

(7) **Synapse**: The space where the nervous impulse jumps from one neuron to another is called the synapse.

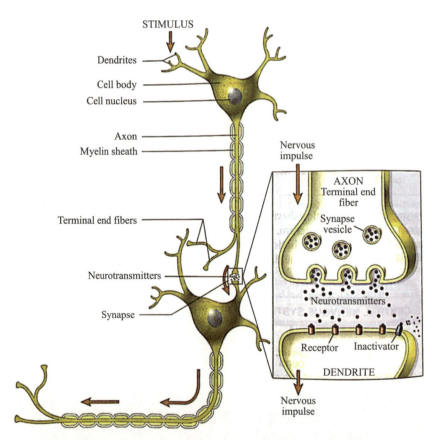

Figure 6-2 Parts of a Neuron and the Pathway of a Nervous Impulse

The stromal tissue of the central nervous system consists of the **glial (neuroglial) cells**, which make up its supportive framework and help it ward off infection. Glial cells do not transmit impulses. They are far more numerous than neurons and can reproduce. There are four types of supporting or glial cells (Figure 6-3).

• **Astrocytes** (**astroglial cells**) are star-like in appearance (*-astr/o* means star) and transport water and salts between capillaries and neurons.

• **Microglial cells** are small cells with many branching processes (dendrites). As phagocytes, they protect neurons in response to inflammation.

• **Oligodendroglial cells** (**oligodendrocytes**) have few (*-olig/o* means few or scanty) dendrites. These cells form the myelin sheath in the CNS.

• **Ependymal cells** (Greek ependyma means upper garment) line membranes within the brain and spinal cord where cerebrospinal fluid (CSF) is produced and circulates.

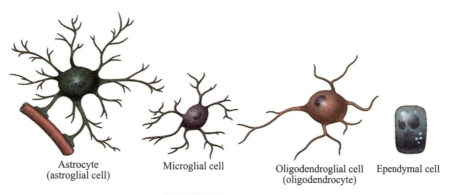

Figure 6-3 Glial Cells

NERVES

Individual neuron fibers are held together in bundles like wires in a cable. If this bundle is part of the **PNS**, it is called a nerve. A collection of cell bodies along the pathway of a nerve is a **ganglion**. A few nerves (sensory nerves) contain only sensory neurons, and a few (motor nerves) contain only motor neurons, but most contain both types of fibers and are described as mixed nerves.

THE BRAIN

The brain is nervous tissue contained within the cranium. It consists of the **cerebrum**, **diencephalon**, **brainstem**, and **cerebellum**. The cerebrum is the largest part of the brain; it is composed largely of white matter with a thin outer layer of gray matter, the **cerebral cortex**. It is within the cortex that the higher brain functions of memory, reasoning, and abstract thought occur. The cerebrums distinct surface is formed by grooves, or **sulci**, and raised areas, or **gyri** (singular: gyrus), that provide additional surface area. The cerebrum is divided into two hemispheres by a deep groove, the longitudinal fissure. Each hemisphere is further divided into lobes with specialized functions. The lobes are named for the skull bones under which they lie

(Figure 6-4).

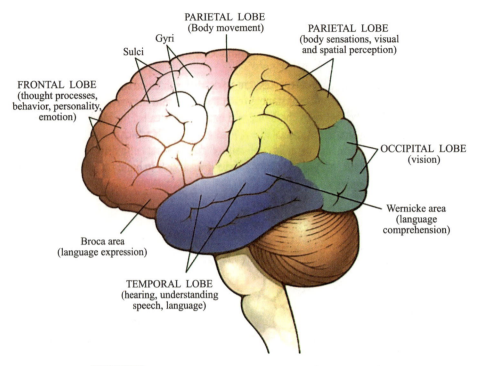

Figure 6-4　External Surfaces of the Brain (lateral view)

The remaining parts of the brain are as follows:

The diencephalon contains the **thalamus**, the **hypothalamus**, and the pituitary gland. The thalamus receives sensory information and directs it to the proper portion of the cortex. The hypothalamus controls the pituitary and forms a link between the endocrine system and nervous system.

The brainstem consists of the:

Midbrain, which contains reflex centers for improved vision and hearing.

Pons, which forms a bulge on the anterior surface of the brainstem. It contains fibers that connect the brain's different regions.

Medulla oblongata, which connects the brain with the spinal cord. All impulses passing to and from the brain travel through this region. The medulla also has vital centers for control of heart rate, respiration, and blood pressure.

The cerebellum is under the cerebrum and dorsal to the pons and medulla oblongata. Like the cerebrum, it is divided into two hemispheres. The cerebellum helps control voluntary muscle movements and to maintain posture, coordination, and balance.

Figure 6-5 shows parts of the brain. Note the location of the pituitary gland below the hypothalamus. The basal ganglia (a group of cells) regulate intentional movements of the body. The corpus callosum lies in the center of the brain and connects the two hemispheres (halves).

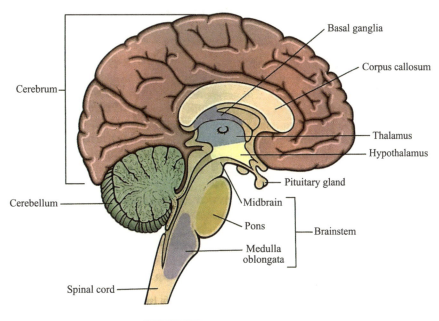

Figure 6-5 Parts of the Brain

PROTECTING THE BRAIN

Within the brain are four **ventricles** (cavities) in which **cerebrospinal fluid** (CSF) is formed. This fluid circulates around the brain and spinal cord, acting as a protective cushion for these tissues.

Covering the brain and the spinal cord are three protective layers, together called the **meninges**. The meninges and adjacent tissue are shown in Figure 6-6. All are named with the Latin word "mater", meaning "mother" to indicate their protective function. They are the:

- **Dura mater**, the outermost and toughest of the three. "Dura" means "hard".
- **Arachnoid mater**, the thin, web-like middle layer. It is named for the Latin word for spider, because it resembles a spider web.
- **Pia mater**, the thin, vascular inner layer, attached directly to the tissue of the brain and spinal cord. "Pia" means "tender".

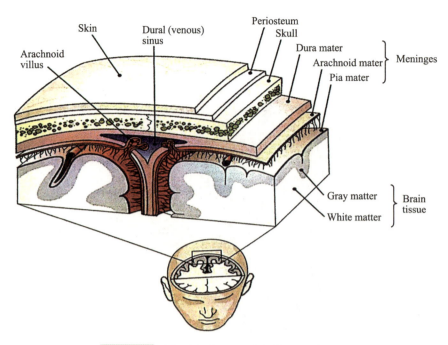

Figure 6-6 The Meninges and Adjacent Tissue

Twelve pairs of **cranial nerves** (Table 6-1 and Figure 6-7) connect with the brain. These nerves are identified by Roman numerals and also by name.

Table 6-1 The Cranial Nerves

NUMBER	NAME	FUNCTION
I	Olfactory	Carries impulses for the sense of smell
II	Optic	Carries impulses for the sense of vision
III	Oculomotor	Controls movement of eye muscles
IV	Trochlear	Controls a muscle of the eyeball
V	Trigeminal	Carries sensory impulses from the faces; controls chewing muscles
VI	Abducent	Controls a muscle of the eyeball
VII	Facial	Controls muscles of facial expression, salivary glands, and tear glands; conducts some impulses for taste
VIII	Vestibulocochlear	Conducts impulses for hearing and equilibrium; also called auditory or acoustic nerve
IX	Glossopharyngeal	Conducts sensory impulses from tongue and pharynx; stimulates parotid salivary gland and partly controls swallowing
X	Vagus	Supplies most organs of thorax and abdomen; controls digestive secretions
XI	Accessory	Controls muscles of the neck
XII	Hypoglossal	Controls muscles of the tongue

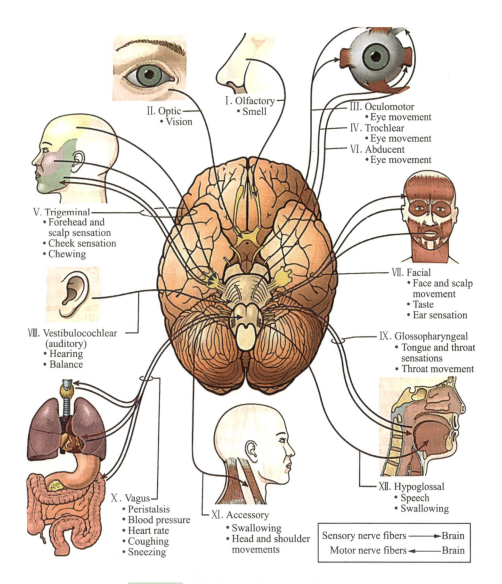

Figure 6-7　The Cranial Nerves (inferior view)

THE SPINAL CORD

The spinal cord begins at the medulla oblongata and tapers to an end between the first and second lumbar vertebrae. It has enlargements in the cervical and lumbar regions, where nerves for the arms and legs join the cord cross section. The spinal cord has a central area of gray matter surrounded by white matter. The gray matter projects toward the posterior and anterior dorsal and ventral horns. The white matter contains the ascending and descending **tracts** (fiber bundles) that carry impulses to and from the brain. A central canal contains CFS.

THE SPINAL NERVES

Thirty-one pairs of **spinal nerves** connect with the spinal cord (Figure 6-8). These nerves are grouped in the segments of the cord as follows:

- Cervical nerves: 8
- Thoracic nerves: 12
- Lumbar nerves: 5
- Sacral nerves: 5
- Coccygeal nerve: 1

Each nerve joins the cord by two roots. The dorsal, or posterior root carries sensory impulses into the cord; the ventral, or anterior root carries motor impulses away from the cord and out toward a muscle or gland. An enlargement on the dorsal root, the dorsal root ganglion, has the cell bodies of sensory neurons carrying impulses toward the CNS.

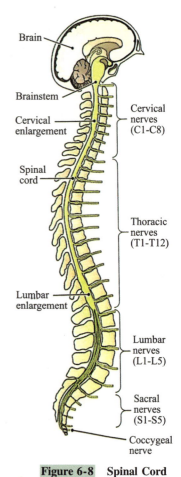

Figure 6-8 Spinal Cord

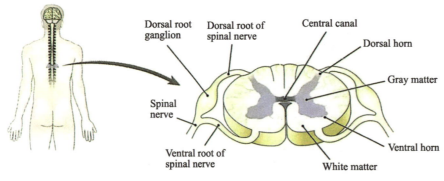

A. Diagram shows the organization of gray and white matter and the roots of the spinal nerves

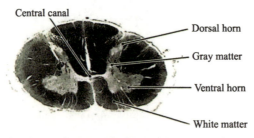

B. Microscopic view of the spinal cord in cross section

Figure 6-9 Spinal Cord, Cross Section

REFLEXES

A simple response that requires few neurons is a **reflex**. In a spinal reflex, impulses travel through the spinal cord only and do not reach the brain. An example of this type of response is the knee-jerk reflex used in physical examinations. The patellar (knee-jerk) reflex is shown in Figure 6-10, with numbers indicating the sequence of impulses. Most neurologic responses, however, involve complex interactions among multiple neurons in the CNS.

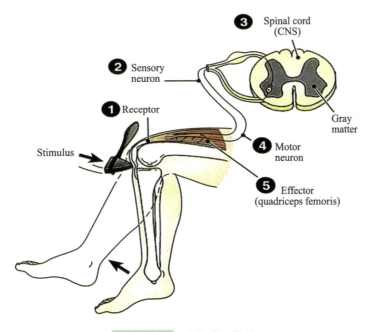

Figure 6-10 A Reflex Pathway

THE AUTONOMIC NERVOUS SYSTEM

The **autonomic nervous system** (ANS) is the division of the nervous system that regulates the involuntary actions of muscles and glands. The ANS itself has two divisions (Figure 6-11).

(1) The **sympathetic nervous system** motivates our response to stress, the so-called fight-or-flight response. It increases heart rate and respiration rate, stimulates the adrenal gland, and delivers more blood to skeletal muscles.

(2) The **parasympathetic nervous system** returns the body to a steady state and stimulates maintenance activities such as digestion of food.

Most organs are controlled by both systems, and in general, the two systems have opposite effects on a given organ.

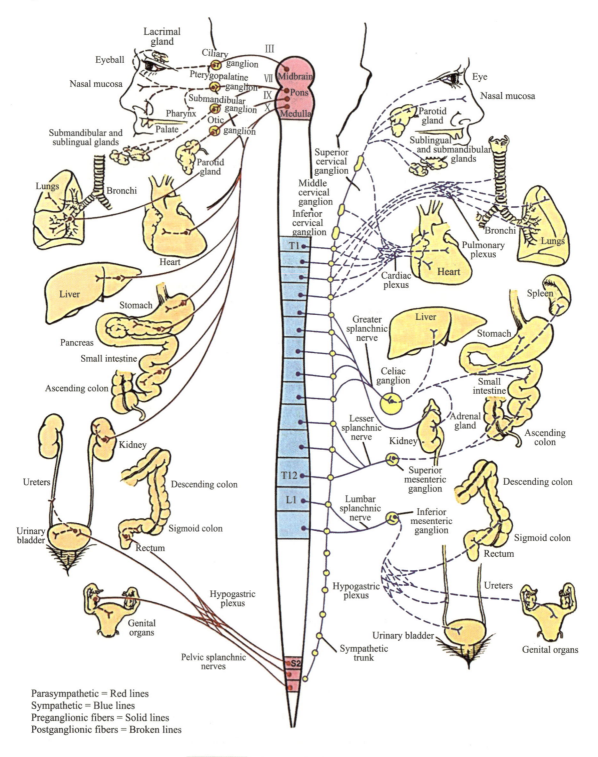

Figure 6-11 Autonomic Nervous System

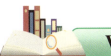

Vocabulary

afferent	/ˈæfərənt/	adj.	传入的
arachnoid mater	/əˈræknɔɪd ˈmeɪtə/		蛛网膜
autonomic nervous system (ANS)	/ˌɔːtəʊˈnɒmɪk ˈnɜːvəs ˈsɪstəm/		自主神经系统
axon	/ˈæksɒn/	n.	轴突
brain	/breɪn/	n.	脑
brainstem	/ˈbreɪnstem/	n.	脑干
central nervous system (CNS)	/ˈsentrəl ˈnɜːvəs ˈsɪstəm/		中枢神经系统
cerebellum	/ˌserəˈbeləm/	n.	小脑
cerebral cortex	/ˈserəbrəl ˈkɔːteks/		大脑皮质
cerebrum	/səˈriːbrəm/	n.	大脑
cerebrospinal fluid (CSF)	/ˌserɪbrəʊˈspaɪnəl ˈfluːɪd/		脑脊液
cranial nerve	/ˈkreɪniəl nɜːv/		颅神经
dendrite	/ˈdendraɪt/	n.	树突
diencephalon	/ˌdaɪenˈsefəlɒn/	n.	间脑
dura mater	/ˈdjʊrə ˈmeɪtə/		硬脑膜
efferent	/ˈefərənt/	adj.	传出的
ganglion	/ˈɡæŋɡliən/	n.	神经节
gray matter	/ɡreɪ ˈmætə/		灰质
gyrus	/ˈdʒaɪrəs/	n.	脑回(复数:gyri)
hypothalamus	/ˌhaɪpəˈθæləməs/	n.	下丘脑
interneuron	/ˌɪntəˈnjʊərɒn/	n.	中间神经元
medulla oblongata	/mɪˈdʌlə ɒblɒŋˈɡɑːtə/		延髓
meninges	/məˈnɪndʒiːz/	n.	脑(脊)膜
midbrain	/ˈmɪdbreɪn/	n.	中脑
myelin	/ˈmaɪəlɪn/	n.	髓鞘;髓鞘质
neuroglia	/njʊəˈrɒɡliə/	n.	神经胶质(细胞)
neuron	/ˈnjʊərɒn/	n.	神经元
neurotransmitter	/ˈnjʊərəʊtrænzmɪtə/	n.	神经递质
parasympathetic nervous system	/ˌpærəˌsɪmpəˈθetɪk ˈnɜːvəs ˈsɪstəm/		副交感神经系统
peripheral nervous system (PNS)	/pəˈrɪf(ə)rəl ˈnɜːvəs ˈsɪstəm/		周围神经系统

pia mater	/ˈpaɪə ˈmeɪtə/		软脑膜
pons	/pɒnz/	n.	脑桥
reflex	/ˈriːfleks/	n.	反射
sensory	/ˈsensəri/	adj. n.	感觉的；感官的 感觉器官
somatic nervous system	/səʊˈmætɪk ˈnɜːvəs ˈsɪstəm/		躯体神经系统
spinal cord	/ˈspaɪnl kɔːd/		脊髓
spinal nerves	/ˈspaɪnl nɜːv/		脊神经
sulcus	/ˈsʌlkəs/	n.	脑沟
synapse	/ˈsɪnæps/	n.	（神经元的）突触
sympathetic nervous system	/ˌsɪmpəˈθetɪk ˈnɜːvəs ˈsɪstəm/		交感神经系统
thalamus	/ˈθæləməs/	n.	丘脑
tract	/trækt/	n.	束
ventricle	/ˈventrɪkl/	n.	脑室
white matter	/waɪt ˈmætə/		白质
visceral nervous system	/ˈvɪsərəl ˈnɜːvəs ˈsɪstəm/		内脏神经系统

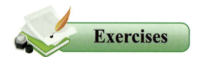

Exercises

I *Match the following terms with their meaning.*

1. _____（1）myelin　　　　　　a. region that connects the brain and spinal cord
   _____（2）diencephalon　　　b. part of the brain that contains the thalamus and pituitary
   _____（3）ganglion　　　　　c. whitish material that covers some axons
   _____（4）medulla oblongata　d. rounded area on the ventral surface of the brainstem
   _____（5）pons　　　　　　　e. collection of neuron cell bodies

2. _____（1）amyloid　　　　　a. accumulation of CFS in the brain
   _____（2）aphasia　　　　　　b. excessive fear of pain
   _____（3）hydrocephalus　　　c. substance associated with Alzheimer disease
   _____（4）paranoia　　　　　d. mental disorder associated with delusions of persecution
   _____（5）odynophobia　　　e. loss of speech communication

3. _____（1）aneurysm　　　　　a. partial paralysis or weakness
   _____（2）convulsion　　　　b. paralysis of the bladder
   _____（3）meningomyelocele　c. series of violent, involuntary muscle contractions

_____(4) paresis   d. localized dilation of a blood vessel
_____(5) cystoplegia   e. hernia of the meninges and spinal cord

Supplementary Terms

4. _____(1) plexus   a. network
   _____(2) corpus callosum b. area of skin supplied by a spinal nerve
   _____(3) dermatome   c. a neurotransmitter
   _____(4) acetylcholine   d. a band of connecting fibers in the brain
   _____(5) ictus   e. a sudden blow or attack

5. _____(1) lethargy   a. fear of being enclosed
   _____(2) ataxia   b. state of sluggishness
   _____(3) claustrophobia c. loss of memory
   _____(4) euphoria   d. lack of muscle coordination
   _____(5) amnesia   e. sense of elation

6. _____(1) PTSD   a. type of psychoactive drug
   _____(2) SSRI   b. system that maintains wakefulness
   _____(3) DSM   c. mental disturbances that follow trauma
   _____(4) RAS   d. degenerative
   _____(5) CJD   e. reference for diagnosis of mental disorders

II *Examine the following statements. If the statement is true, write "T" in the blank. If the statement is false, write "F" in the blank.*

_____ 1. Sensory fibers conduct impulses toward the CNS.

_____ 2. CSF forms in the ventricles of the brain.

_____ 3. The cervical nerves are in the region of the neck.

_____ 4. Myelinated neurons make up the gray matter of the CNS.

_____ 5. The spinal nerves are part of the central nervous system.

_____ 6. The fiber that carries impulses toward the neuron cell body is the axon.

_____ 7. There are 12 pairs of cranial nerves.

_____ 8. The outermost layer of the meninges is the pia mater.

_____ 9. Hyperlexia refers to increased skills in reading.

III *Match the name with each numbered part and write the number in the corresponding blank.*

1. ANATOMIC DIVISIONS OF THE NERVOUS SYSTEM

_____ Brain

_____ Central nervous system

_____ Cranial nerves

_____ Peripheral nervous system

_____ Spinal cord

_____ Spinal nerves

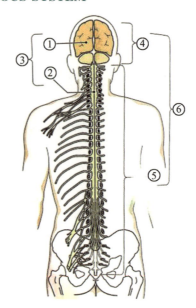

2. MOTOR NEURON

_____ Axon branch

_____ Muscle

_____ Myelin

_____ Nucleus

_____ Axon covered with sheath

_____ Cell body

_____ Dendrites

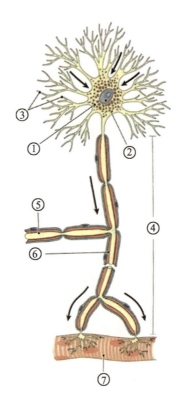

3. EXTERNAL SURFACE OF THE BRAIN

_____ Cerebellum

_____ Frontal lobe

_____ Gyri

_____ Medulla oblongata

_____ Occipital lobe

_____ Parietal lobe

_____ Pons

_____ Spinal cord

_____ Sulci

_____ Temporal lobe

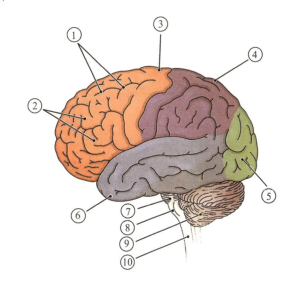

4. SPINAL CORD, LATERAL VIEW

_____ Brain

_____ Brainstem

_____ Cervical enlargement

_____ Cervical nerves

_____ Coccygeal nerve

_____ Lumbar enlargement

_____ Lumbar nerves

_____ Sacral nerves

_____ Spinal cord

_____ Thoracic nerves

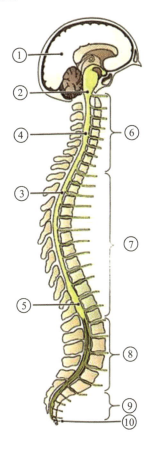

5. SPINAL CORD, CROSS SECTION

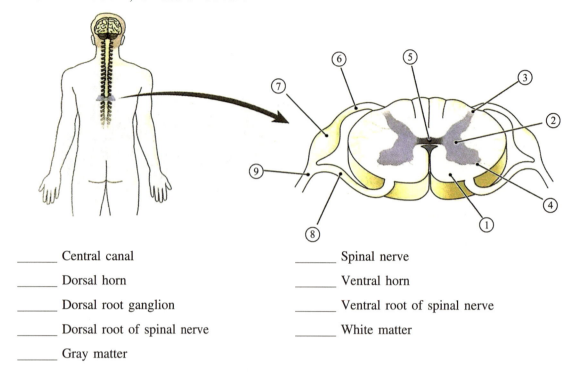

_____ Central canal

_____ Dorsal horn

_____ Dorsal root ganglion

_____ Dorsal root of spinal nerve

_____ Gray matter

_____ Spinal nerve

_____ Ventral horn

_____ Ventral root of spinal nerve

_____ White matter

6. REFLEX PATHWAY

_____ Effector

_____ Motor neuron

_____ Receptor

_____ Sensory neuron

_____ Spinal cord (CNS)

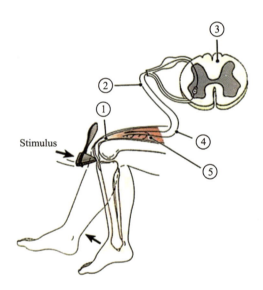

CHAPTER 7

CIRCULATORY SYSTEM
循环系统

Chapter Sections

- Introduction
- Cardiovascular system
- Lymphatic system
- Anatomy of the heart
- Vocabulary
- Exercises

Chapter Goals

- To describe the structure of the heart.
- To trace the pathway of blood through the heart.
- To list the functions and components of the lymphatic system.
- To describe the location of the heart and its four chambers.

INTRODUCTION

Blood circulates throughout the body in the **cardiovascular system**, which consists of the heart and the blood vessels. This system forms a continuous circuit that delivers oxygen and nutrients to all cells and carries away waste products. The **lymphatic system** also functions in circulation. Its vessels drain fluid and proteins left in the tissues and return them to the **bloodstream**. The lymphatic system plays a part in immunity and in the digestive process as well.

CARDIOVASCULAR SYSTEM

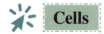

Cells

Body cells are dependent on a constant supply of nutrients and oxygen. When the supplies are delivered and then chemically combined, they release the energy necessary to do the work of each cell. How does the body ensure that oxygen and food will be delivered to all of its cells? The cardiovascular system, consisting of the heart(a powerful muscular pump) and blood vessels (fuel line and transportation network) performs this important work.

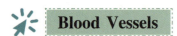

Blood Vessels

There are three types of blood vessels in the body: **arteries**, **veins** and **capillaries.**

Arteries are large blood vessels that carry blood away from the heart. Their walls are lined with connective tissue, muscle tissue, and elastic fibers, with an innermost layer of epithelial cells called **endothelium**. Endothelial cells, found in all blood vessels, secrete factors that affect the size of blood vessels, reduce blood clotting, and promote the growth of blood vessels. Because arteries carry blood away from the heart, they must be strong enough to withstand the high pressure of the pumping action of the heart. Their elastic walls allow them to expand as the heartbeat forces blood into the arterial system throughout the body.

Smaller branches of arteries are **arterioles**. Arterioles are thinner than arteries and carry the blood to the tiniest of blood vessels, the capillaries.

Capillaries have walls that are only one endothelial cell in thickness. These delicate, microscopic vessels carry nutrient-rich, oxygenated blood from the arteries and arterioles to the body cells. Their thin walls allow passage of oxygen and nutrients out bloodstream and into cells. There, the nutrients are burned in the presence of oxygen (catabolism) to release energy. At the same time, waste products such as carbon dioxide and water pass out of cells and into the thin-walled capillaries. Waste-filled blood then flows back to the heart in small **venules**, which combine to form larger vessels called veins.

Veins have thinner walls compared with arteries. They conduct blood (that has given up most of its oxygen) toward the heart from the tissues. Veins have little elastic tissue and less connective tissue than that typical of arteries, and blood pressure in veins is extremely low compared with pressure in arteries. In order to keep blood moving back toward the heart, veins have **valves** that prevent the backflow of blood and keep the blood moving in one direction. Muscular action also helps the movement of blood in veins.

Circulation of Blood

Arteries, arterioles, veins, venules, and capillaries, together with the heart, form a circulatory system for the flow of blood. Figure 7-1 is a more detailed representation of the entire circulatory system. Refer to it as you read the following paragraphs. (Note that the bracketed numbers in the following paragraphs correspond with those in Figure 7-1.)

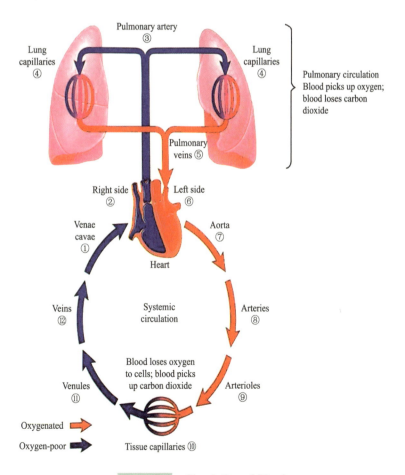

Figure 7-1 **Circulation of Blood**

Figure 7-2 shows the aorta, selected arteries, and pulse points. The **pulse** is the beat of the heart as felt through the walls of arteries.

Blood that is deficient in oxygen flows through two large veins, the **venae cavae**① on its way from the tissue capillaries to the heart. The blood becomes oxygen-poor at the tissue capillaries when oxygen leaves the blood and enters the body cells.

Oxygen-poor blood enters the **right side of the heart**② and travels through that side and into the **pulmonary artery**③, a vessel that divides in two: one branch leading to the left lung, the other to the right lung. The arteries continue dividing and subdividing within the lungs, forming smaller and smaller vessels (arterioles) and finally reaching the **lung capillaries** ④. The pulmonary artery is unusual in that it is the only artery in the body that carries blood deficient in oxygen.

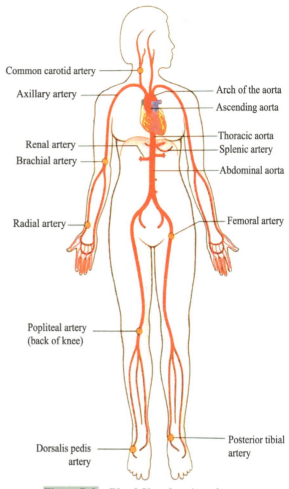

Figure 7-2 Blood Vessels—Arteries

While passing through the lung (pulmonary) capillaries, blood absorbs the oxygen that entered the body during inhalation. The newly oxygenated blood next returns immediately to the heart through **pulmonary veins**⑤. The pulmonary veins are unusual in that they are the only veins in the body that carry oxygen-rich (oxygenated) blood. The circulation of blood through the vessels from the heart to the lungs and then back to the heart again is the pulmonary circulation.

Oxygen-rich blood enters the **left side of the heart** ⑥ from the pulmonary veins. The muscles in the left side of the heart pump the blood out of the heart through the largest single artery in the body—the **aorta** ⑦. The aorta moves up at first (ascending aorta) but then arches over dorsally and runs downward (descending aorta) just in front of the **vertebral column.** The aorta divides into numerous branches called **arteries**⑧ that carry the oxygenated blood to all parts of the body. The names of some of these arterial branches will be familiar to you: brachial (brachi/o means arm), axillary, splenic, gastric, and renal arteries. The carotid arteries supply blood to the head and neck.

The relatively large arterial vessels branch further to form smaller **arterioles** ⑨. The arterioles, still containing oxygenated blood, branch into smaller **tissue capillaries** ⑩, which are near the body cells. Oxygen leaves the blood and passes through the thin capillary walls to enter the body cells. There, food is broken down, in the presence of oxygen, and energy is released.

This chemical process also releases carbon dioxide (CO_2), as a waste product. Carbon dioxide passes out from the cell into the tissue capillaries at the same time that oxygen enters. Thus the blood returning to the heart from tissue capillaries, through **venules** ⑪ and **veins** ⑫ is filled with carbon dioxide but is depleted of oxygen.

As this oxygen-poor blood enters the heart from the venae cavae, the circuit is complete. The pathway of blood from the heart to the tissue capillaries and back to the heart is the **systemic circulation**.

LYMPHATIC SYSTEM

Lymph

Lymph is a clear, watery fluid that surrounds body cells and flows in a system of thin-walled lympha vessels (the lymphatic system) that extends throughout the body.

Lymph differs from blood, but it has a close relationship to the blood system. Lymph fluid does not contain **erythrocytes** or **platelets**, but it is rich in two types of white blood cells (**leukocytes**): **lymphocytes** and **monocytes**. The liquid part of lymph is similar to blood plasma in that it contains water, salts, sugar, and wastes of metabolism such as **urea** and **creatinine**, but it differs in that it contains less protein. Lymph actually originates from the blood. It is the same fluid that filters out of tiny blood capillaries into the spaces between cells. This fluid that surrounds body cells is called interstitial fluid. Interstitial fluid passes continuously into specialized thin-walled vessels called lymphatic capillaries, which are found coursing through tissue spaces. The fluid in the lymphatic capillaries, now called lymph instead of interstitial fluid, passes through larger lymphatic vessels and through clusters of lymph tissues (lymph nodes), finally reaching large lymphatic vessels in the upper chest. Lymph enters these large lymphatic vessels, which then empty into the bloodstream.

Functions

The lymphatic system has several functions.

First, it is a drainage system to transport needed proteins and fluid that have leaked out of the blood capillaries (and into the interstitial fluid) back to the bloodstream via the veins.

Second, the lymphatic vessels in the intestines absorb lipids (fats) from the small intestine and transport them to the bloodstream.

A third function of the lymphatic system relates to the immune system: the defense of the body against foreign **organisms** such as bacteria and viruses. Lymphocytes and monocytes, originating in bone marrow, lymph nodes, and organs such as the spleen and thymus gland, protect the body by producing antibodies and by mounting a cellular attack on foreign cells and organisms.

ANATOMY OF THE HEART

The human heart weighs less than a pound, is roughly the size of an adult fist, and lies in the thoracic cavity, just behind the breastbone in the mediastinum (between the lungs).

The heart is a pump consisting of four chambers: two upper chambers called **atria** (singular: atrium) and two lower chambers called **ventricles**. It is actually a double pump, bound into one organ and synchronized very carefully. Blood passes through each pump in a definite pattern. Pump station number one, on the right side of the heart, sends oxygen-deficient blood to the lungs, where the blood picks up oxygen and releases its carbon dioxide. The newly oxygenated blood returns to the left side of the heart to pump station number two and does not mix with the oxygen-poor blood in pump station number one. Pump station number two then forces the oxygenated blood out to all parts of the body. At the body tissues, the blood loses its oxygen, and on returning to the heart, to pump station number one, blood poor in oxygen (rich in carbon dioxide) is sent out to the lungs to begin the cycle anew.

Oxygen-poor blood enters the heart through the two largest veins in the body, the **venae cavae**. The superior vena cava drains blood from the upper portion of the body, and the inferior vena cava carries blood from the lower part of the body.

The venae cavae bring oxygen-poor blood that has passed through all of the body to the right atrium, the thin-walled upper right chamber of the heart. The right atrium contracts to force blood through the **tricuspid valve** (cusps are the flaps of the valves) into the right ventricle, the lower right chamber of the heart. The cusps of the tricuspid valve form a one-way passage designed to keep the blood flowing in only one direction. As the right ventricle contracts to pump oxygen-poor blood through the pulmonary valve into the pulmonary artery, the tricuspid valve stays shut, thus preventing blood from pushing back into the right atrium. The pulmonary artery then branches to carry oxygen-deficient blood to each lung.

The blood that enters the lung capillaries from the pulmonary artery soon loses its large quantity of carbon dioxide into the lung tissue, and the carbon dioxide is expelled. At the same time, oxygen enters the capillaries of the lungs and is brought back to the heart via the pulmonary veins. The newly oxygenated blood enters the left atrium of the heart from the pulmonary veins. The walls of the left atrium contract to force blood through the mitral valve into the left ventricle.

The left ventricle has the thickest walls of all four heart chambers (three times the thickness of the right ventricular wall). It must pump blood with great force so that the blood travels through arteries to all parts of the body. The left ventricle propels the blood through the aortic valve into the aorta, which branches to carry blood all over the body. The aortic valve closes to prevent return of aortic blood to the left ventricle.

Figure 7-3 shows the pathway of blood through the heart.

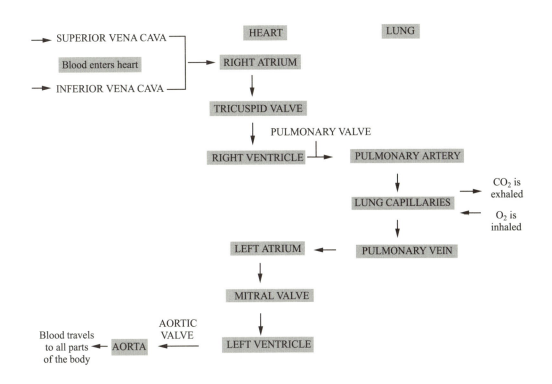

Figure 7-3   Pathway of Blood Through the Heart

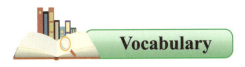

aorta	/eɪˈɔːrtə/	n.	主动脉
arteriole	/ɑːrˈtɪəriəʊl/	n.	小动脉
artery	/ˈɑːrtəri/	n.	动脉
atrium (plural : atria)	/ˈeɪtriəm/	n.	心房
capillary	/ˈkæpəleri/	n.	毛细血管
carbon dioxide (CO_2)	/ˌkɑːrbən daɪˈɒksaɪd/	n.	二氧化碳
diastole	/daɪˈæstəli/	n.	心脏舒张;心脏舒张期
endothelium	/ˌendəʊˈθiːliəm/	n.	内皮
mitral valve	/ˈmaɪtrəl vælv/	n.	左房室瓣(二尖瓣)
oxygen	/ˈɒksɪdʒən/	n.	氧,氧气
pulmonary artery	/ˈpʌlmənəri ˈɑːrtəri/		肺动脉
pulmonary circulation	/ˈpʌlmənəri ˌsɜːrkjəˈleɪʃn/		肺循环
pulmonary valve	/ˈpʌlmənəri vælv/		肺动脉瓣
pulmonary vein	/ˈpʌlmənəri veɪn/		肺静脉

septum (plural: septa)	/ˈseptəm/	n.	隔膜
systemic circulation	/sɪˈstemɪk ˌsɜːrkjəˈleɪʃn/		体循环
systole	/ˈsɪstəli/	n.	心脏收缩,心缩期
tricuspid valve	/traɪˈkʌspəd vælv/		三尖瓣
valve	/vælv/	n.	瓣膜
vein	/veɪn/	n.	静脉
vena cava (plural: venae cavae)	/ˌviːnə ˈkeɪvə/		腔静脉
ventricle	/ˈventrɪkl/	n.	室;心室;脑室
venule	/ˈvenjuːl/	n.	小静脉

Exercises

I *Choose from the listed structures for each of the descriptions that follow.*

aorta	inferior vena cava	superior vena cava
arteriole	mitral valve	tricuspid valve
atrium	pulmonary artery	ventricle
capillary	pulmonary vein	venule

1. valve that lies between the right atrium and the right ventricle: _____

2. the smallest blood vessel: _____

3. it carries oxygenated blood from the lungs to the heart: _____

4. the largest artery in the body: _____

5. it brings oxygen-poor blood into the heart from the upper parts of the body: _____

6. upper chamber of the heart: _____

7. it carries oxygen-poor blood to the lungs from the heart: _____

8. small artery: _____

9. valve that lies between the left atrium and the left ventricle: _____

10. it brings blood from the lower half of the body to the heart: _____

11. small vein: _____

12. lower chamber of the heart: _____

II *Trace the path of blood through the heart. Begin as the blood enters the right atrium from the venae cavae (and include the valves within the heart).*

1. right atrium
2. _____
3. _____
4. _____
7. _____
8. _____
9. _____
10. _____

5. _____   11. _____
6. capillaries of the lung   12. _____

III *Complete the following sentences with proper terms.*

1. The wall of the heart between the right and the left atria is the _____.
2. The relaxation phase of the heartbeat is called _____.
3. Specialized conductive tissue in the wall between the ventricles is the _____.
4. The inner lining of the heart is the _____.
5. The contractive phase of the heartbeat is called _____.
6. A gas released as a metabolic product of catabolism is _____.

IV *Complete the following terms using the given definitions.*

1. surgical repair of a valve: valvulo _____
2. condition of deficient oxygen: hyp _____
3. pertaining to an upper heart chamber: _____ al
4. narrowing of the mitral valve: mitral _____
5. breakdown of a clot: thrombo _____

CHAPTER 8

THE ICF: AN OVERVIEW
ICF概论

Chapter Sections

Introduction

Aims

Underlying principles

The ICF model

ICF components and their contents

Applying ICF for rehabilitation management

Vocabulary

Exercises

Chapter Goals

- To understand how ICF is applied in rehabilitation.

INTRODUCTION

The International Classification of Functioning, Disability and Health (ICF) is a framework for describing and organizing information on functioning and disability. It provides a standard language and a conceptual basis for the definition and measurement of health and disability.

The ICF was approved for use by the World Health Assembly in 2001, after extensive testing across the world involving people with disabilities and people from a range of relevant disciplines. A companion classification for children and youth (ICF-CY) was published in 2007.

The ICF integrates the major models of disability. It recognizes the role of environmental factors in the creation of disability, as well as the relevance of associated health conditions and their effects.

This overview provides a brief introduction to the ICF—its structure, contents, purposes and applications.

AIMS

The ICF is a multipurpose classification system designed to serve various disciplines and sectors—for example in education and transportation as well as in health and community services—and across different countries and cultures.

The aims of the ICF are to:

· provide a scientific basis for understanding and studying health and health-related states, outcomes, determinants, and changes in health status and functioning;

· establish a common language for describing health and health-related states in order to improve communication between different users, such as health care workers, researchers, policy-makers and the public, including people with disabilities;

· permit comparison of data across countries, health care disciplines, services and time;

· provide a systematic coding scheme for health information systems.

The ICF has been accepted as one of the United Nations social classifications and provides an appropriate instrument for the implementation of stated international human rights mandates as well as national legislation. Therefore, the ICF provides a valuable framework for monitoring aspects of the "UN Convention on the Rights of Persons with Disabilities" (UN 2006), as well as for national and international policy formulation.

UNDERLYING PRINCIPLES

Four general principles guide the development of the ICF and are essential to its application.

Universality. A classification of functioning and disability should be applicable to all people irrespective of health condition and in all physical, social and cultural contexts. The ICF achieves this and acknowledges that anyone can experience some disability. It concerns everyone's functioning and disability, and was not designed, nor should be used, to label persons with disabilities as a separate social group.

Parity and aetiological neutrality. In classifying functioning and disability, there is not an explicit or implicit distinction between different health conditions, whether "mental" or "physical". In other words, disability is not differentiated by aetiology. By shifting the focus from health condition to functioning, it places all health conditions on an equal footing, allowing them to be compared using a common metric. Further, it clarifies that we cannot infer participation in everyday life from diagnosis alone.

Neutrality. Domain definitions are worded in neutral language, wherever possible, so that the classification can be used to record both the positive and negative aspects of functioning and disability.

Environmental Influence. The ICF includes environmental factors in recognition of the important role of environment in people's functioning. These factors range from physical factors (such as climate, terrain or building design) to social factors (such as attitudes, institutions, and laws). Interaction with environmental factors is an essential aspect of the scientific understanding of "functioning and disability".

THE ICF MODEL

In the ICF, functioning and disability are multi-dimensional concepts, relating to:

· the body functions and structures of people, and impairments thereof (functioning at the level of the body);

· the activities of people (functioning at the level of the individual) and the activity limitations they experience;

· the participation or involvement of people in all areas of life, and the participation restrictions they experience (functioning of a person as a member of society);

· the environmental factors which affect these experiences (and whether these factors are facilitators or barriers).

The ICF conceptualizes a person's level of functioning as a dynamic interaction between her or his health conditions, environmental factors, and personal factors. It is a biopsychosocial model of disability, based on an integration of the social and medical models of disability.

As illustrated in Figure 8-1, disability is multidimensional and interactive. All components of disability are important and any one may interact with another. Environmental factors must be taken into consideration as they affect everything and may need to be changed.

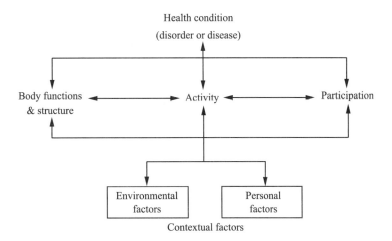

Figure 8-1 Interactions Between the Components of ICF

ICF COMPONENTS AND THEIR CONTENTS

The major components of functioning and disability are understood "in the context of health" which clarifies that participation restrictions related to other factors, such as racial prejudice, are not within the scope of the ICF. Table 8-1 explains terms used in ICF.

Table 8-1　Explanation of Terms used in ICF

Body functions	The physiological functions of body systems (including psychological functions).
Body structures	Anatomical parts of the body such as organs, limbs and their components.
Impairments	Problems in body function and structure such as significant deviation or loss.
Activity	The execution of a task or action by an individual.
Participation	Involvement in a life situation.
Activity limitations	Difficulties an individual may have in executing activities.
Participation restrictions	Problems an individual may experience in involvement in life situations.
Environmental factors	The physical, social and attitudinal environment in which people live and conduct their lives. These are either barriers to or facilitators of the person's functioning.
Functioning	An umbrella term for body function, body structures, activities and participation. It denotes the positive or neutral aspects of the interaction between a person's health condition(s) and that individual's contextual factors (environmental and personal factors).
Disability	An umbrella term for impairments, activity limitations and participation restrictions. It denotes the negative aspects of the interaction between a person's health condition(s) and that individual's contextual factors (environmental and personal factors).

Each component contains hierarchically arranged domains. These are sets of related physiological functions, anatomical structures, actions, tasks, areas of life, and external influences. The ICF has a separate chapter for each of the domains as listed in Table 8-2.

Table 8-2 ICF Components and Domains/Chapters

ICF Components	Domains/Chapters
Body Function	Mental functions
	Sensory functions and pain
	Voice and speech functions
	Functions of the cardiovascular, haematological, immunological and respiratory systems
	Functions of the digestive, metabolic, endocrine systems
	Genitourinary and reproductive functions
	Neuromusculoskeletal and movement-related functions
	Functions of the skin and related structures
Body Structure	Structure of the nervous system
	The eye, ear and related structures
	Structures involved in voice and speech
	Structure of the cardiovascular, immunological and respiratory systems
	Structures related to the digestive, metabolic and endocrine systems
	Structure related to genitourinary and reproductive systems
	Structures related to movement
	Skin and related structures
Activities and Participation	Learning and applying knowledge
	General tasks and demands
	Communication
	Mobility
	Self care
	Domestic life
	Interpersonal interactions and relationships
	Major life areas
	Community, social and civic life
Environmental Factors	Products and technology
	Natural environment and human-made changes to environment
	Support and relationships
	Attitudes
	Services, systems and policies

APPLYING ICF FOR REHABILITATION MANAGEMENT

Rehabilitation aims to enable people experiencing or likely to experience disability to achieve and maintain optimal functioning. It is the starting point of a patient and goal oriented rehabilitation process. With the ICF rehabilitation practitioners can rely for the first on a worldwide accepted model providing a universal language for the description and classification of functioning.

To take advantage of the ICF in rehabilitation management there is a need to develop appropriate ICF tools for clinical practice. Such ICF tools, integrating the model and classification of the ICF, have to be integrated in a problem solving approach provided by the Rehab-Cycle. ICF tools have been developed for the use in the different steps of the Rehab-Cycle.

In rehabilitation management ICF Core Sets serve as a guide to comprehensively assess and describe functioning. To quantify the extent of a problem, facilitator or barrier in the different ICF categories of ICF Core Sets, the ICF also comprises ICF Qualifiers. A problem may mean an impairment restriction, which can be qualified from 0(No barrier), 1(Mild barrier), 2(Moderate barrier), 3(Severe barrier), 4(Complete barrier). Environmental factors are qualified with a negative and positive scale that denotes the extent to which an environmental factor acts as a barrier or a facilitator.

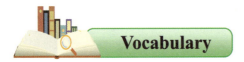

Vocabulary

activity	/ækˈtɪvəti/	n.	（个体）活动
body functions and structure			身体功能和结构
cardiovascular	/ˌkɑːdiəʊˈvæskjələ/	adj.	心血管的
disability	/ˌdɪsəˈbɪləti/	n.	残疾
domestic life	/dəˈmestɪk/		日常生活
genitourinary	/ˌdʒenɪtəʊˈjʊərɪnərɪ/	adj.	泌尿系统的
handicap	/ˈhændikæp/	n.	残障
impairment	/ɪmˈpeəmənt/	n.	（身体或智力方面的）缺陷,障碍,损伤
immunological and respiratory systems	/ˌɪmjʊnəˈlɒdʒɪkl/ /ˈrespərətɔːri/		免疫和呼吸道系统
metabolic	/ˌmetəˈbɒlɪk/	adj.	新陈代谢的
participation	/pɑːˌtɪsɪˈpeɪʃn/	n.	参加,参与

The International Classification of Functioning, Disability and Health (ICF)			国际功能、残疾和健康分类
universality	/ˌjuːnɪvɜːˈsælətɪ/	n.	普遍性

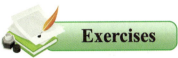

Draw the figure of interactions between the components of ICF in this frame.

CHAPTER 9

PHYSICAL THERAPY
物理治疗

Chapter Sections

Introduction

Definition

Category

History

Education

Development

Vocabulary

Exercises

Chapter Goals

- To define physical therapy.
- To describe the characteristics of physical therapy.
- To identify the development and history of the physical therapy profession.
- To be familiar with basic medical terminology.

INTRODUCTION

Physical therapy (PT) attempts to address the illnesses, or injuries that limit a person's abilities to move and perform functional activities in their daily lives.

Physical therapists (PTs) use an individual's history and physical examination to arrive at a diagnosis and establish a management plan and, when necessary, incorporate the results of laboratory and imaging studies like X-rays, CT-scan, or MRI findings. Electrodiagnostic testing may also be used.

PT management commonly includes prescription of or assistance with specific exercises, manual therapy and manipulation, mechanical devices such as traction, education, physical agents which includes heat, cold, electricity, sound waves, radiation, assistive devices, prostheses, orthoses and other interventions.

In addition, PTs work with individuals to prevent the loss of mobility before it occurs by developing fitness and wellness-oriented programs for healthier and more active lifestyles, providing services to individuals and populations to develop, maintain and restore maximum movement and functional ability throughout the lifespan. This includes providing therapeutic treatment in circumstances where movement and function are threatened by aging, injury, disease or environmental factors. Functional movement is central to what it means to be healthy.

Physical therapy is a professional career which has many specialties including musculoskeletal, sports, neurology, wound care, EMG, cardiopulmonary, geriatrics, orthopedics, women's health, and pediatrics. Neurological rehabilitation is in particular a rapidly emerging field.

PTs practice in many settings, such as private-owned physical therapy clinics, outpatient clinics or offices, health and wellness clinics, rehabilitation hospitals facilities, skilled nursing facilities, extended care facilities, private homes, education and research centers, schools, hospices, industrial and this workplaces or other occupational environments, fitness centers and sports training facilities.

Physical therapists also practise in the non-patient care roles such as health policy, health insurance, health care administration and as health care executives. Physical therapists are involved in the medical-legal field serving as experts, performing peer review and independent medical examinations.

DEFINITION

Physical therapy (PT), also known as **physiotherapy**, is one of the allied health professions that, by using functional training, manual therapy and physical agents which include heat, cold, water, electricity, sound waves, radiation, mechanical force, remediate impairments and promote mobility and function.

Physical therapy is used to improve a patient's quality of life through examination, diagnosis, prognosis, physical intervention, and patient education. It is performed by **physical therapists** (known as **physiotherapists in many countries**).

In addition to clinical practice, other activities encompassed in the physical therapy profession include research, education, consultation and administration. Physical therapy services may be provided as primary care treatment or alongside, or in conjunction with, other medical services.

CATEGORY

Physical therapy can be divided into three categories: functional training, manual therapy and physical agents.

Functional training mainly includes muscle strength training, transfer training, balance and coordination training, and walking training.

Manual therapy uses skills such as joint mobilization, stretching, NPT (neurophysiological therapy), PNF (proprioceptive neuromuscular facilitation), motor learning and CIMT (constrained-included movement therapy).

Physical agents includes electrotherapy, phototherapy, ultrasound therapy, magnetotherapy, hydrotherapy, BFT (biofeedback therapy), paraffin therapy, hypothermia, compression therapy and traction.

HISTORY

Physicians like Hippocrates and later Galenare are believed to have been the first practitioners of physical therapy, advocating massage, manual therapy techniques and hydrotherapy to treat people in 460 BC.

The history of modern physical therapy was traced from its origins in World War I. The poliomyelitis and the World War I increased the number of disabled people, which called for rapid advances in physical therapy. In the decades after World War II, growth and development were paramount features of the profession. In the past ten years, with the rise of modern science, physical therapy has been continuously developed and improved.

EDUCATION

Educational criteria for physical therapy providers vary from country to country, and among various levels of professional responsibility. Most countries have licensing bodies that require physical therapists to be a member of before they can start practicing as independent professionals.

DEVELOPMENT

Telehealth (or telerehabilitation) is a developing form of physical therapy in response to the increasing demand for physical therapy treatment. Telehealth is online communication between the clinician and patient, either live or in pre-recorded sessions. The benefits of telehealth include improved accessibility in remote areas, cost efficiency, and improved convenience for the bedridden and home-restricted, physically disabled. Some considerations for telehealth include: limited evidence to prove effectiveness and compliance more than in-person therapy, licensing and payment policy issues, and compromised privacy. Studies are controversial as to the effectiveness of telehealth in patients with more serious conditions, such as stroke, multiple sclerosis, and lower back pain.

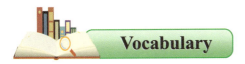

Vocabulary

physiotherapy	/ˌfɪziəʊˈθerəpi/	n.	物理疗法；理疗
physiotherapist	/ˌfɪziəʊˈθerəpɪst/	n.	物理疗法医师；理疗师
traction	/ˈtrækʃn/	n.	牵引
electrodiagnostic testing	/ɪˌlektrəʊdaɪəɡˈnɒstɪk/		电诊断测验
functional training	/ˈfʌŋkʃənl ˈtreɪnɪŋ/		功能训练
manual therapy	/ˈmænjuəl ˈθerəpi/		手法治疗
joint mobilization	/dʒɔɪnt ˌməʊbɪlaɪˈzeɪʃn/		关节松动
stretching	/ˈstretʃɪŋ/	n.	拉伸肌肉
NPT (neurophysiological therapy)	/ˌnjʊərəʊfɪziˈɒlədʒi ˈθerəpi/		神经生理学疗法

PNF (proprioceptive neuromuscular facilitation)	/ˌprəʊprɪə(ʊ)ˈseptɪv ˌnjʊərəʊˈmʌskjələ fəˌsɪlɪˈteɪʃn/		本体神经肌肉促进技术
motor learning	/ˈməʊtə ˈlɜːnɪŋ/		运动再学习技术
CIMT (constrained-included movement therapy)	/kənˈstreɪnd ɪnˈkluːdɪd ˈmuːvmənt ˈθerəpi/		强制性使用运动治疗
physical agent	/ˈfɪzɪkl ˈeɪdʒənt/		物理因子疗法
electrotherapy	/ɪˌlektrəˈθerəpi/	n.	电疗法
phototherapy	/ˌfəʊtəˈθerəpi/	n.	光疗法
ultrasound therapy	/ˈʌltrəsaʊnd ˈθerəpi/		超声疗法
magnetotherapy	/mæɡˌniːtəʊˈθerəpi/	n.	磁疗法
hydrotherapy	/ˌhaɪdrəʊˈθerəpi/	n.	水疗法
BFT (biofeedback therapy)	/ˌbaɪəʊˈfiːdbæk ˈθerəpi/		生物反馈疗法
paraffin therapy	/ˈpærəfɪn ˈθerəpi/		石蜡疗法
hypothermia therapy	/ˌhaɪpəˈθɜːmiə ˈθerəpi/		低温疗法
compression therapy	/kəmˈpreʃn ˈθerəpi/		压力疗法
telehealth	/ˈtelɪhelθ/	n.	远程医疗

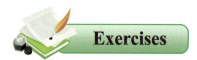

Exercises

I *Answer the following questions.*

1. What is the definition of physical therapy and physical therapist?
2. What are the physical therapists doing to get the patient's diagnosis?
3. What does a physical therapist do with a patient?
4. What is the category of physical therapy?
5. When does modern physical therapy originate?
6. What is telehealth and what is the advantage of it?

II *Judge whether the following statements are true (T) or false (F).*

1. A physiotherapist can only work in a hospital.
2. Physical therapists can make their plans without communicating with patients.
3. A physical therapist can work without a license.
4. Physical therapy can serve cardiopulmonary rehabilitation.
5. PTs can arrive at a diagnosis and establish a management plan by incorporating the results of laboratory and imaging studies.
6. Muscle strength training is a skill of manual therapy.
7. The origin of modern physical therapy is due to the prevalence of the poliomyelitis.

8. Telehealth is a service that physiotherapists need to go to the patient's home.

9. The benefits of telehealth include improved accessibility in remote areas, more effective and compliant, and improved convenience for the bedridden and home-restricted, physically disabled.

III *Reading comprehension.*

Communication in Physical Therapy in the Twenty-First Century

Physical therapy practitioners of the twenty-first century agree that communication is integral to the successful practice of physical therapy.

PTs are professionals who use a variety of professional communication behaviors that may enhance their effectiveness in the clinical and educational settings. Several research studies indicate that communication is one of the most important skills used by physical therapy professionals. Communication skills include the ability to listen, read, and write effectively. They also include effective verbal and nonverbal skills in interactions with clients, families, colleagues, supervisors, and support staff. Cultural, verbal, and behavioral rapport skills can be learned and implemented in the classroom and the clinic to enhance communication effectiveness.

Strategies are discussed for communicating effectively with diverse groups, including:

- Individuals who come from cultures different from your own
- Individuals who speak little or no English
- Individuals who come from a generation different from your own
- Individuals who have visual impairments
- Individuals who have hearing impairments
- Patients/clients and caregivers
- Health care team members
- Support staff
- Faculty and clinical supervisors
- Those who use digital communication

Students first learn these professional communication behaviors in their physical therapy classes and apply the behaviors with their faculty and peers. By practicing these behaviors during classroom experiences, students are better prepared to develop them as they proceed from beginning skills as students to post-entry-level skills as they become physical therapy providers.

CASE STUDIES

• CASE STUDY ONE

You are a PT student working in an early intervention program in Miami, Florida. You have been assigned to evaluate a 2-year-old boy with Down syndrome whose family recently immigrated to Miami from Nicaragua. The family is very concerned because their son is not yet walking. You do not speak Spanish, and you are expected to complete the evaluation with the child and the family. What professional behaviors will you use to enhance your communication with this family?

Tips

1. Request a bicultural and bilingual medical interpreter for the examination and evaluation.
2. Use your behavioral rapport skills with the family when the interpreter is translating.
3. Speak with cultural informants in your clinical setting who are knowledgeable about Nicaraguan culture.
4. Seek written or web resources to learn more about Nicaraguan culture.
5. Learn essential physical therapy phrases in Spanish to help you communicate verbally with the family in subsequent treatment sessions.
6. Contact your CI for assistance if the family has difficulty understanding your examination, evaluation, or intervention suggestions.

• CASE STUDY TWO

You are a PT or PTA student completing your clinical internship at an inpatient rehabilitation hospital. Your CI has given you feedback at your midterm evaluation that your nonverbal communication indicates that you are disinterested and aloof when working with patients. You are upset because you were not aware that you were conveying disinterest or aloofness toward patients. Your CI stated that she observed you standing about 10 feet away from her patients with your arms folded across your chest when she was treating them. She stated that other staff members had noticed similar nonverbal patterns when you observed their patient treatments. What professional behaviors will you use to enhance your communication in this situation?

Tips

1. Meet with your CI and ask for specific constructive feedback related to your nonverbal behaviors. Explain that you had not realized how your nonverbal behavior had been perceived.
2. Take responsibility for the behavior and indicate your willingness to modify your behavior appropriately.
3. Contact the academic coordinator of clinical education (ACCE) at your institution and request her assistance in remediation for your nonverbal skills.
4. Complete a self-assessment of your communication and interpersonal skills using the generic abilities.
5. Meet with your CI and the ACCE to compare your self-assessment with the assessment of your nonverbal communication by the CI.
6. Develop a plan for modifying your nonverbal behavior with the assistance of the CI and the ACCE.
7. Modify your behavior by implementing your verbal and behavioral rapport skills.
8. Meet with your CI and ACCE to evaluate your new behavior after a week.

CHAPTER 10

OCCUPATIONAL THERAPY
作业治疗

Chapter Sections

What is occupational therapy?

What does occupational science mean?

Is occupational therapy the same as physical therapy?

Where do occupational therapists work?

Who should study occupational therapy?

What are the outcomes?

Vocabulary

Exercises

Chapter Goals

- To understand what is occupational therapy.
- To know how occupational therapists work.

WHAT IS OCCUPATIONAL THERAPY?

In its simplest terms, occupational therapists and occupational therapy assistants help people of all ages participate in the things they want and need to do through the therapeutic use of everyday activities (occupations). Unlike other professions, occupational therapy helps people function in all of their environments (e.g., home, work, school, community) and addresses the physical, psychological, and cognitive aspects of their well-being through engagement in occupation.

Common occupational therapy interventions include helping children with disabilities participate fully in school and develop social skills, helping people recovering from injury regain function through retraining and/or adaptations, and providing supports for older adults experiencing physical and cognitive changes. Occupational therapy services typically include:

- an **individualized evaluation**, during which the client, family, and occupational therapist determine the person's goals,
- **customized intervention**, to improve the person's ability to perform daily activities and reach the goals, and
- an **outcomes evaluation**, to ensure that the goals are being met and/or to modify the intervention plan based on the patient's needs and skills.

Occupational therapy services may include comprehensive evaluations of the client's home and other environments, recommendations for adaptive equipment and training in its use, training in how to modify a task or activity to facilitate participation, and guidance and education for family members and caregivers. Entry-level practice requires a master's degree for occupational therapists and an associate's degree for occupational therapy assistants (who must be supervised by an OT).

WHAT DOES OCCUPATIONAL SCIENCE MEAN?

Occupational science is a new discipline that provides the basic science information about "occupations" or activities that support the practice of occupational therapy. Occupational science studies how activities meet the needs of individuals and communities and provide meaning and purpose to life; how activities produce changes in the individual and different patterns of occupation. This is similar to how sociology is applied in social work, and biology applied in medicine.

IS OCCUPATIONAL THERAPY THE SAME AS PHYSICAL THERAPY?

No, they are not the same. The physical therapist usually focuses on the movement of the body, while the occupational therapist helps people of all ages (from newborns to older adults) who have an illness or disability do those things that are important and meaningful to them such as eating, dressing, school activities, and work. The occupational therapist helps by making changes in any of the things that may limit an individual's ability to do those tasks, including the environment, the task, or the person's skills needed for the task. Occupational therapists also have the knowledge and training to work with people with a mental illness or emotional problems such as depression and/or stress.

WHERE DO OCCUPATIONAL THERAPISTS WORK?

Occupational therapists work in a variety of settings. These could include hospitals, rehabilitation centers, nursing facilities, home health, outpatient clinics, private practice, school systems, private organizations, industry, and community agencies such as return to work programs, prisons, and community settings. The number of different places where therapists work is growing every year.

WHO SHOULD STUDY OCCUPATIONAL THERAPY

Occupational therapy is a challenging and fascinating job combining creativity and problem solving with the ability to make practical, meaningful changes in a person's life. As an occupational therapist, you will use your knowledge, critical thinking, and hands-on skills to help others. Since occupational therapists work intensely with people, good personal skills such as good communication skills, an interest and commitment to serving or helping other people, and an interest in social and biological sciences are also helpful.

WHAT ARE THE OUTCOMES?

Occupational therapy is a science-driven profession that applies the most up-to-date research to service delivery. Evidence supports the effectiveness of adding an occupational therapy practitioner to your patients or clients treatment plan. According to systematic reviews from AOTA's (American Occupational Therapy Association) "Evidence-Based Practice Occupational Therapy Practice Guidelines", evidence shows that the following occupational therapy interventions improve client outcomes. These interventions are used as part of a broad approach that considers the patient's performance skills (motor, process, social interaction); activity demands; performance patterns (habits, routines, rituals, roles); and contexts and environments.

Pediatrics

1. Early Childhood

- Play-based activities, rehearsal of social behaviors, modeling, and prompting to improve social behaviors;
- Oral stimulation programs, skin-to-skin contact, and sensory-motor-oral interventions to reduce the length of hospital stay;
- An early intervention program for preterm infants to improve cognitive outcomes in infancy and preschool;
- Infant massage to improve sleep and relaxation, reduce crying, and reduce hormones affecting stress;
- A caregiver-delivered home program for infants updated at 1, 2, and 3 months to improve motor performance;
- Family-centered help-giving that incorporates support to strengthen the family to improve satisfaction, parenting behavior, personal and family well-being, social support, and child behavior.

2. Mental Health

- Social and life skills programs for children with intellectual impairments and developmental delays to improve life skills, conversation turn-taking, initiation of social interaction, self-management, and compliance, and to decrease problem behaviors;
- Parenting programs for teenage mothers and their children to improve mother-infant interaction and parental attitudes and knowledge, maternal mealtime communication, self-confidence, and identity;
- Structured recreation and activity program for children with extreme shyness to increase extraversion and decrease timidity.

3. Sensory Integration and Sensory Processing

- A cognitive and task-based approach to address participation in occupations for children with motor-deficits characteristic of Developmental Coordination Disorder (DCD);

● Sensory integration for gross motor and motor planning skills for children with learning disabilities;

● Sensory integration to address maladaptive behaviors in children with problems in sensory processing;

● Touch pressure/deep pressure and massage to address touch aversion and improved responsiveness to sound in children with autism.

Gerontology

● Client-centered occupational therapy to improve physical functioning and occupational performance related to health management in frail older adults, and older adults with osteoarthritis and macular degeneration;

● Home modification and adaptive equipment provided by occupational therapy practitioners to reduce functional decline and improve safety;

● Exercise involving functional activities for older adults;

● Progressive resistance strength training to improve community mobility and meal preparation. Strengthening, balance retraining, and a walking plan to reduce falls and injuries for those older than 80 years;

● Short-term classroom and on-road instruction to improve driving knowledge and skills;

● Use of bioptics to improve simulated and on-road driving skills as well as outdoor mobility skills for older adults with visual impairments.

Rehabilitation & Disability

● Inpatient rehabilitation for individuals with multiple sclerosis to reduce disease severity and improve ADL status;

● Home-based, individualized, and computerized cognitive training to improve attention, memory, information processing, and executive functions for individuals with multiple sclerosis;

● Multi-session, repetitive physical exercise tasks for individuals with Parkinson disease to improve diachronic motor and sensory-perceptual performance skills;

● Client-preferred external cues during ADLs to improve motor control for individuals with disabilities.

Parkinson Disease

● Multidisciplinary program to improve survival, increase the use of appropriate assistive devices, and facilitate a higher quality of life in social functioning and mental health;

● Therapy based on personally meaningful tasks to increase therapeutic gains for individuals recovering from stroke;

● Instructions that focus on task-related parameters rather than on specific movement-related parameters, to improve movement organization among stroke survivors;

- Brief program of occupational therapy in home following discharge from hospital after stroke to improve recovery;
- Occupational therapy in stroke survivors' homes focusing on community mobility, to increase community participation;
- Practice dressing for stroke survivors to improve independence in dressing and maintain improvements after therapy.

Adults with Serious Mental Illnesses

- Life and social skills training with extended training in natural environments, to improve daily interactions;
- Cognitive skills training in conjunction with supported employment to improve job retention;
- Lifestyle interventions to improve health behaviors related to obesity and metabolic syndrome to reduce health care costs;
- Supported education programs to meet postsecondary education goals to promote independence;
- Physical activity, exercise, and outdoor activities to improve symptoms of depression and anxiety;
- Social cognition and problem solving training to enhance community participation.

Work

- Client-centered approaches, rather than predetermined regimens, to reduce disability and improve function, including return to work;
- Therapeutic occupations and activities, rather than bed rest, to reduce pain and improve functional recovery for individuals with low back pain;
- Meaningful and relevant therapeutic hand activities combining multiple movement patterns, force, and volition to facilitate better outcomes than exercise alone.

Vocabulary

participate	/pɑːˈtɪsɪpeɪt/	vi.	参加;参与
profession	/prəˈfeʃn/	n.	职业,专业;同行;宣称
psychological	/ˌsaɪkəˈlɒdʒɪkl/	adj.	心理的,精神上的,精神(现象)的;心理学(上)的,关于心理学的
well-being	/ˈwel biːɪŋ/	n.	健康,安乐;康乐
retraining	/ˌriːˈtreɪnɪŋ/	n.	再培训;再教育

adaptation	/ˌædæpˈteɪʃn/	n.	适应,顺应;改编,改编本
individualized evaluation			个性化评价
client	/ˈklaɪənt/	n.	顾客;当事人;诉讼委托人
customized intervention			个性化干预
outcomes evaluation			结果评估
comprehensive	/ˌkɒmprɪˈhensɪv/	adj.	全部的,所有的,(几乎)无所不包的,详尽的;综合性的
facilitate	/fəˈsɪlɪteɪt/	vt.	促进,促使,使便利
caregiver	/ˈkeəɡɪvə(r)/	n.	照料者,护理者
entry-level	/ˈentri levəl/	adj.	适用于初学者的,初级的
associate	/əˈsəʊʃieɪt/	vt.	联想,联系;交往
newborn	/ˈnjuːbɔːn/	adj.	(婴儿)新生的,初生的
depression	/dɪˈpreʃn/	n.	抑郁症;抑郁,沮丧;下陷处,坑;经济衰退,不景气
outpatient	/ˈaʊtpeɪʃnt/	n.	门诊病人,不住院病人
Alzheimer's disease			阿尔茨海默病
cerebral palsy			脑瘫
autism	/ˈɔːtɪzəm/	n.	孤独症
limb	/lɪm/	n.	肢,臂,腿,翅膀
hands-on	/ˌhændzˈɒn, -ˈɔːn/	adj.	亲自实践的;实际动手操作的
science-driven		adj.	科学带领的
pediatrics	/ˌpiːdɪˈætrɪks/	n.	小儿科;儿科学;幼科
rehearsal	/rɪˈhɜːsl/	n.	排练,排演;彩排,演习;复述,详述
stimulation	/ˌstɪmjʊˈleɪʃn/	n.	刺激;激发;启发;促进
preterm infant	/ˌpriːˈtɜːm ˈɪnfənt/		早产儿
preschool	/ˈpriːskuːl/	n.	幼儿园
hormone	/ˈhɔːməʊn/	n.	荷尔蒙,激素
incorporate	/ɪnˈkɔːpəreɪt/	vt.	将……包括在内,包含,吸收;使并入
impairment	/ɪmˈpeəmənt/	n.	损害,损伤
compliance	/kəmˈplaɪəns/	n.	服从,顺从,遵从
integration	/ˌɪntɪˈɡreɪʃn/	n.	结合,整合,一体化;(不同肤色、种族、宗教信仰等的人的)混合,融合
Developmental Coordination Disorder			发育性共济失调
osteoarthritis	/ˌɒstiəʊɑːˈθraɪtɪs/	n.	骨关节炎

macular	/ˈmækjʊlə/	adj.	有斑点的,有污点的
degeneration	/dɪˌdʒenəˈreɪʃn/	n.	退化,衰退,堕落
bioptic	/baɪˈɒptɪk/	adj.	活组织检查的
sclerosis	/skləˈrəʊsɪs/	n.	硬化症
Parkinson disease			帕金森病
diachronic	/ˌdaɪəˈkrɒnɪk/	adj.	探求现象变化的,历时的
multidisciplinary	/ˌmʌltidɪsəˈplɪnəri/	adj.	包括各种学科的,涉及多学科的
parameter	/pəˈræmɪtə(r)/	n.	决定因素,规范,范围
conjunction	/kənˈdʒʌŋkʃn/	n.	连词;结合,同时发生
maternal	/məˈtɜːnl/	adj.	母亲的,母亲般的;母系的,母亲方面的
obesity	/əʊˈbiːsəti/	n.	肥胖,过胖;肥胖症
metabolic	/ˌmetəˈbɒlɪk/	adj.	新陈代谢的;变化的
syndrome	/ˈsɪndrəʊm/	n.	综合征,综合症状;典型表现
postsecondary		n.	高等教育
predetermine	/ˌpriːdɪˈtɜːmɪn/	vt.	预先决定,事先安排

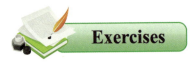

Exercises

I *Describe the daily work of an occupational therapist in the hospital.*

_____
_____
_____
_____
_____
_____
_____

II *What kind of patients do the occupational therapists focus on?*

_____
_____
_____
_____
_____
_____
_____

III *What can an occupational therapist do about Parkinson disease?*

CHAPTER 11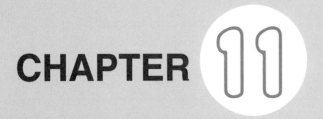

SPEECH AND LANGUAGE REHABILITATION
言语康复

Chapter Sections

Introduction

The types of disorders

The therapy area

The case

Commentary

Vocabulary

Exercises

Chapter Goals

- To distinguish the speech and language.
- To master the different disorders about the speech.
- To know the general situation of speech rehabilitation.

INTRODUCTION

Speech-language pathology is a field of expertise practiced by a clinician known as a **speech-language pathologist** (**SLP**), also sometimes referred to as a **speech and language therapist** or a **speech therapist**. SLP is considered a "related health profession" along with audiology, optometry, occupational therapy, clinical psychology, physical therapy, and others. The field of SLP is distinguished from other related health professions as SLPs are legally permitted to diagnose certain disorders which fall within their scope of practice. SLPs specialize in the evaluation, diagnosis, and treatment of **communication disorders** (speech disorders and language disorders), **cognitive-communication disorders**, **voice disorders**, and **swallowing disorders**. SLPs also play an important role in the diagnosis and treatment of autism spectrum disorder (often in a team with pediatricians and psychologists).

THE TYPES OF DISORDERS

A common misconception is that speech-language pathology is restricted to adjusting a speaker's speech sound articulation to meet the expected normal pronunciation, such as helping English speaking individuals enunciate the traditionally difficult "r". SLPs can also often help people who stutter speak more fluently. Articulation and fluency are only two facets of the work of an SLP, however. In fact, speech-language pathology is concerned with a broad scope of speech, language, swallowing, and voice issues involved in communication, some of which include:

- Word-finding and other semantic issues, either as a result of a **specific language impairment** (**SLI**) such as a language delay or as a secondary characteristic of a more general issue such as dementia.
- Social communication difficulties involving how people communicate or interact with others (pragmatics).
- Structural language impairments, including difficulties in creating sentences that are grammatical (syntax) and modifying word meaning (morphology).
- Literacy impairments (reading and writing) related to the letter-to-sound relationship (phonics), the word-to-meaning relationship (semantics), and understanding the ideas presented in a text (reading comprehension).
- Voice difficulties, such as a raspy voice, a voice that is too soft, or other voice difficulties that negatively impact a person's social or professional performance.

- Cognitive impairments (e.g., attention, memory, executive function) to the extent that they interfere with communication.

Speech is the spoken production of language and the process through which sounds are produced. The components of speech production include:

- phonation (producing sound),
- resonance,
- fluency,
- intonation,
- pitch variance,
- voice (including aeromechanical components of respiration).

Language is a system used to represent thoughts and ideas. Language is made up of several rules that explain what words mean, how to make new words, and how to put words together to form sentences. The components of language include:

- phonology (manipulating sound according to the rules of a language),
- morphology (understanding components of words and how they can modify meaning),
- syntax (constructing sentences according to the grammatical rules of a target language),
- semantics (interpreting signs or symbols of communication such as words or signs to construct meaning),
- pragmatics (social aspects of communication).

Primary pediatric speech and language disorders include: receptive and expressive language disorders, speech sound disorders, childhood apraxia of speech (CAS), stuttering, and language-based learning disabilities. Speech pathologist not only work with adolescents with speech and language impediments, but also those that are elderly.

Swallowing disorders include difficulties in any system of the swallowing process (i.e. oral, pharyngeal, esophageal), as well as functional dysphagia and feeding disorders. Swallowing disorders can occur at any age and can stem from multiple causes.

THE THERAPY AREA

Speech-language pathologists (SLPs) provide a wide range of services, mainly on an individual basis, as support for individuals, families, support groups, and providing information for the general public. SLPs work to prevent, assess, diagnose, and treat speech, language, social communication, cognitive-communication, and swallowing disorders in children and adults. Speech services begin with initial screening for communication and swallowing disorders and continue with assessment and diagnosis, consultation for the provision of advice regarding management, intervention, and treatment, and providing counseling and other follow up services for these disorders. Services are provided in the following areas:

- cognitive aspects of communication attention, memory, problem-solving, executive functions;
- speech phonation, articulation, fluency, resonance, and voice including aeromechanical components of respiration (the speech disorders such as apraxia of speech dysarthria and stuttering);
- language (phonology, morphology, syntax, semantics, and pragmatic/social aspects of communication) including comprehension and expression in oral, written, graphic, and manual modalities; language processing; preliteracy and language-based literacy skills, phonological awareness (the language disorders such as aphasia, specific language impairment);
- swallowing or other upper aerodigestive functions such as infant feeding and aeromechanical events (evaluation of esophageal function is for the purpose of referral to medical professionals);
- voice (hoarseness, dysphonia), poor vocal volume (hypophonia), abnormal (e. g. rough, breathy, strained) vocal quality (Research demonstrates voice therapy to be especially helpful with certain patient populations; individuals with Parkinson disease often develop voice issues as a result of their disease.);
- sensory awareness related to communication, swallowing, or other upper aerodigestive functions.

Speech, language, and swallowing disorders result from a variety of causes, such as a stroke, brain injury, hearing loss, developmental delay, a cleft palate, cerebral palsy, or emotional issues.

THE CASE

A 68-year-old woman was hospitalized after awakening one morning unable to speak and with right-sided weakness.

Speech evaluation the next day demonstrated normal oral movements with the exception of limited tongue excursion to the right. She produced only off-target groping movements of her jaw and lips when asked to clear her throat, click her tongue, blow or whistle. Her reflexive cough was normal. She produced only awkward, groping, off-target jaw and lip movements when asked to count, sing a familiar tune, or imitate simple sounds or syllables. She could produce a distorted /a/, /əʊ/ and /ʊ/ on imitation. She was able to imitate /m/ in isolation but could not imitate other isolated sounds. She achieved correct articulatory place for /f/ but could not simultaneously move air to produce frication.

The neurologic verbal and reading comprehension were normal even for difficult comprehension tasks. Writing with her preferred right hand was awkward because of weakness, but spelling, word choice, and grammar were normal.

CT scan 5 days after onset identified a lesion in the left hemisphere at the junction of the posterior frontal and anterior parietal lobes. The neurologic diagnosis was left hemisphere stroke.

Speech therapy was undertaken. At the time of discharge 6 weeks later, she was producing most sounds within single syllables, although slowly and with syllable segregation when she attempted to string syllables together. When reassessed 2 months later, she was speaking laboriously in sentences, with a moderately slowed rate and segregated syllables, deliberate articulation and pervasive mild articulatory distortions. When reassessed 2 years later, speech was functional but characterized by a moderately slowed rate and occasional articulatory substitutions, especially on multisyllabic words. She had consistent difficulty with /z/ and all consonant clusters.

COMMENTARY

(1) Stroke is the most common cause of AOS (Apraxia Of Speech), and AOS may be the only or most prominent manifestation of stroke.

(2) AOS can be characterized by muteness at onset, although people mute from AOS usually attempt to speak.

(3) Although AOS usually occurs with aphasia, even severe AOS can exist without any evidence of language impairment.

(4) AOS is frequently accompanied by NVOA (Nonverbal Oral Apraxia).

(5) When caused by stroke, AOS tends to improve over time, sometimes dramatically. The prognosis may be best when there is little or no language impairment.

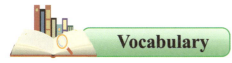

Vocabulary

audiology	/ˌɔːdiˈɒlədʒi/	n.	听力学
optometry	/ɒpˈtɒmətri/	n.	视光学
autism spectrum disorder	/ˈɔːtɪzəm ˈspektrəm dɪsˈɔːdə/		孤独症谱系障碍
articulation	/ɑːˌtɪkjuˈleɪʃn/	n.	说话,吐词,发音
enunciate	/ɪˈnʌnsieɪt/	vt. & vi.	清晰地发(音)
semantic	/sɪˈmæntɪk/	adj.	语义学的
dementia	/dɪˈmenʃə/	n.	痴呆,精神错乱
pragmatics	/præɡˈmætɪks/	n.	语用学
syntax	/ˈsɪntæks/	n.	句法
morphology	/mɔːˈfɒlədʒi/	n.	形态学,形态论;词法,形态学
phonics	/ˈfɒnɪks/	n.	读音教学法,拼读法
executive function	/ɪɡˈzekjətɪv ˈfʌŋkʃn/		执行力
phonation	/fəʊˈneɪʃn/	n.	发声
resonance	/ˈrezənəns/	n.	洪亮,响亮;共振,共鸣,回响
intonation	/ˌɪntəˈneɪʃn/	n.	语调;音准
pitch	/pɪtʃ/	n.	音高
aeromechanical components of respiration	/ˈeərəʊmɪˈkænɪkəl/		呼吸力学组成
phonology	/fəˈnɒlədʒi/	n.	音系,音系学
pharyngeal	/fəˈrɪndʒɪəl/	adj.	咽部的
esophageal	/ˌiːsəˈfædʒɪəl/	adj.	食道的
dysphagia	/dɪsˈfeɪdʒɪə/	n.	吞咽困难
apraxia	/əˈpræksɪə/	n.	失用症
dysarthria	/dɪsˈɑːθrɪə/	n.	构音障碍
stutter	/ˈstʌtə(r)/	vt. & vi.	口吃
aeromechanical	/ˌeərəʊmɪˈkænɪkəl/	adj.	空气力学的
hoarseness	/ˈhɔːsnəs/	n.	嘶哑
dysphonia	/dɪsˈfəʊnɪə/	n.	发声困难

| hypophonia | /haɪpəˈfəʊnɪə/ | n. | 发音过弱 |
| cleft palate | /kleft ˈpælət/ | | 腭裂 |

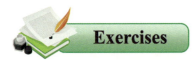

Exercises

Fill in the blanks according to the text.

1. The components of speech production include: _____, _____, _____, _____, _____, _____, _____.

2. The components of language include: _____, _____, _____, _____, _____.

3. Speech-language pathology is concerned with a broad scope of speech, language, swallowing, and voice issues involved in communication, some of which include: _____, _____, _____, _____, _____, _____.

4. The SLPs provide services in the following areas: _____, _____, _____, _____, _____, _____.

CHAPTER 12

PEDIATRIC REHABILITATION
儿童康复

Chapter Sections

History

Definition

Purpose

Cerebral palsy

Management

Vocabulary

Exercises

Chapter Goals

- To become acquainted with terms that describe pediatric rehabilitation.
- To learn to evaluate and diagnose cerebral palsy.
- To understand the treatment's objects and methods of pediatric rehabilitation.

HISTORY

Pediatric rehabilitation has a long history. Rehabilitation physicians began to provide rehabilitation treatment for disabled children in the early 1940s when modern rehabilitation medicine was founded. In 2003, the United States began to establish a pediatric rehabilitation-related certificate management system. In the 1980s, under the leadership of the older generation of pediatric rehabilitation workers led by Professor Li Shuchun, pediatric rehabilitation was introduced into China, and pediatric rehabilitation led by the rehabilitation of cerebral palsy (hereinafter referred to as cerebral palsy) has a history of more than 40 years. In China, pediatric rehabilitation has been expanded from cerebral palsy, which is a disease related to congenital malformations, developmental disorders, autism spectrum disorders, attention deficit hyperactivity disorders, learning disorders, epilepsy, genetic and metabolic diseases, central or peripheral nerve injury, motor injury, rare diseases and other related diseases in children. Rehabilitation for disabled children is also the focus of pediatric rehabilitation. In the 1980s, the rehabilitation of disabled people in China was first incorporated into the national development plan, and the rehabilitation of disabled children began to receive policy support at the national level. Following the five-year plan of national economic and social development, China's rehabilitation work for children has been gradually promoted and perfected with the support of the China Disabled Persons Federation.

DEFINITION

Pediatric rehabilitation is applying medical, educational, social and occupational methods in a comprehensive and coordinated manner to anyone who is under the age of 18, recovering and rebuilding the functions of the sick, the injured and the disabled as soon as possible so that their physical, mental, social and economic abilities can be restored to the greatest extent possible. It aims to enhance and restore functional ability and quality of life to those with physical impairments or disabilities.

PURPOSE

The main aims of pediatric rehabilitation are to promote functional development: gross motor function, fine motor function, perception, language understanding and expression, social ability, mental health, self-care, learning (motor function, language expression, social ability, correction of abnormal posture, abnormal motor patterns, abnormalities) and muscle tension.

CEREBRAL PALSY

Cerebral palsy (**CP**) is a group of permanent movement disorders that appear in early childhood, caused by abnormal development or damage to the parts of the brain that control movement, balance and posture. Most often, the problems occur during pregnancy; however, they may also occur during childbirth or shortly after birth.

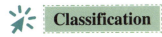
Classification

There are three main cerebral palsy (CP) classifications by motor impairment: **spastic**, **ataxic**, and **athetoid/dyskinetic**. Additionally, there is a mixed type that shows a combination of features of the other types. These classifications reflect the areas of the brain that are damaged. Cerebral palsy is also classified according to the topographic distribution of muscle spasticity. This method classifies children as **diplegic** (bilateral involvement with leg involvement greater than arm involvement), **hemiplegic** (unilateral involvement), or **quadriplegic** (bilateral involvement with arm involvement equal to or greater than leg involvement).

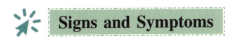
Signs and Symptoms

Cerebral palsy causes activity limitation that is attributed to non-progressive disturbances that occurred in the developing fetal or infant brain. While movement problems are the central feature of CP, difficulties with thinking, learning, feeling, communication and behavior often co-occur.

MANAGEMENT

Physiotherapy (also known as physical therapy) programs are designed to encourage the patient to build a strength base for improved gait and volitional movement, together with stretching programs to limit contractures. Physiotherapists can teach parents how to position and handle their child for activities of daily living.

Speech therapy helps control the muscles of the mouth and jaw, and helps improve communication. Just as CP can affect the way a person moves their arms and legs, it can also affect the way they move their mouth, face and head. This can make it hard for the person to breathe, talk clearly, and bite, chew and swallow food.

Biofeedback (Figure 12-1) is a therapy in which people learn how to control their affected muscles. Biofeedback therapy has been found to significantly improve gait in children with cerebral palsy. Mirror therapy has been used to improve hand function and was found to be generally effective in enhancing muscle strength, motor speed, muscle activity, and the accuracy of both hands.

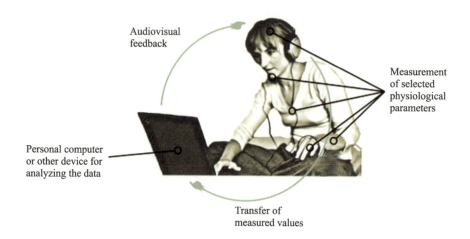

Figure 12-1 Pattern of Biofeedback

Massage therapy is designed to help relax tense muscles, strengthen muscles, and keep joints flexible.

Occupational therapy helps adults and children maximum their function, adapt to their limitations and live as independently as possible. Parents typically enable and support performance of meaningful activities and enable, change and use the environment.

Gait analysis (Figure 12-2) is often used to describe gait abnormalities in children. Gait training has been shown to improve walking speed in children and young adults with cerebral palsy.

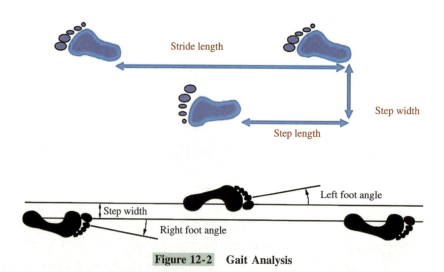

Figure 12-2 Gait Analysis

Medication: Several kinds of medication have been used to treat the various kinds of cerebral palsy.

Cognitive training: **Imitation** is a common way to improve mobility, following three steps:

(1) from gross motor to fine motor;

(2) from fine motor to skilled motor;

(3) combination of motor skills.

Conductive education (CE)

The system has to provide possibilities for children to practice emerging skills not only in specific learning situations but in the many inter-connecting, in-between situations of which life consists. In order to achieve this, CE turns any given part of a child's day into a learning situation.

Sensory integration therapy is based on A. Jean Ayres' Sensory Integration Theory, that describes how the neurological process of processing and integrating sensory information from the body and the environment contribute to emotional regulation, learning, behavior, and participation in daily life, empirically derived disorders of sensory integration and an intervention approach.

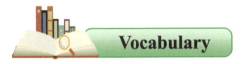

Vocabulary

pediatric rehabilitation	/piːdɪˈætrɪk ˌriːəˌbɪlɪˈteɪʃn/		儿童康复
gross motor	/ɡrəʊs ˈməʊtə(r)/		粗大运动
fine motor	/faɪn ˈməʊtə(r)/		精细运动
cerebral palsy (CP)	/səˈriːbrəl ˈpɔːlzi/		脑瘫
spastic	/ˈspæstɪk/	adj.	痉挛的
ataxic	/əˈtæksɪk/	adj.	共济失调的
athetoid	/ˈæθetəd/	adj.	手足徐动症的
diplegic	/daɪˈpliːdʒɪk/	adj.	双侧瘫痪的
hemiplegic	/heˈmɪpliːdʒɪk/	adj.	偏瘫的
quadriplegic	/ˌkwɑːdrɪˈpliːdʒɪk/	adj.	四肢瘫痪的
gait analysis			步态分析
cognitive training			认知训练
contracture	/kənˈtræktʃə/	n.	挛缩
sensory integration therapy			感觉统合疗法
biofeedback	/ˌbaɪəʊˈfiːdbæk/	n.	生物反馈

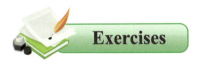

Exercises

1 *Write down the classification of children with cerebral palsy.*

II *Measure your own stride length, step width and step length.*

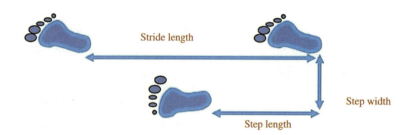

III *Please list at least five treatments for pediatric rehabilitation.*

CHAPTER 13

PSYCHIATRIC REHABILITATION
精神康复

Chapter Sections

- Introduction
- Psychiatric clinical symptoms
- Therapeutic modalities
- Exercises

Chapter Goals

- To describe tests used by clinical psychologists to evaluate a patient's mental health and intelligence.
- To define terms that describe major psychiatric disorders.
- To identify terms that describe psychiatric symptoms.
- To compare different types of therapy for psychiatric disorders.

INTRODUCTION

Some, but not all, psychiatric disorders are not readily explainable in terms of abnormalities in the structure or chemistry of an organ or tissue, as are other illnesses. In addition, the causes of mental disorders are complex and include significant psychological and social as well as chemical and structural elements. This chapter provides a simple outline of psychiatric disorders and definitions of major psychiatric terms.

Psychiatry(psych/o = mind, iatr/o = treatment) is the branch of medicine that deals with the diagnosis, treatment, and prevention of mental illness. It is a specialty of clinical medicine like surgery, internal medicine, pediatrics, and obstetrics.

Clinical psychologists are trained in the use of tests to evaluate various aspects of a patient's mental health and intelligence. Examples are intelligence (IQ) tests such as the Wechsler Adult Intelligence Scale (WAIS) and the Stanford-Binet Intelligence Scale. Two projective (personality) tests are the use of Rorschach Test, in which inkblots, as shown in Figure 13-1, are used to bring out associations, and the Thematic Apperception Test (TAT), in which pictures are used as stimuli for making up stories (Figure 13-2). Both tests are revealing of personality structure. Examples of graphomotor projection tests are the Draw a Person Test, in which the patient is asked to copy a body, and the Bender-Gestalt Test, in which the patient is asked to draw certain geometric designs. The Bender-Gestalt Test picks up deficits in mental processing and memory caused by brain damage and is used to screen children for developmental delays. The Minnesota Multiphasic Personality Inventory (MMPI) contains true-false questions that reveal aspects of personality, such as sense of duty or responsibility, ability to relate to others, and dominance (assertiveness, resourcefulness).

This test is widely used as a measure of psychological health in adolescents and adults. The patient's responses to questions are compared with responses made by patients with diagnoses of schizophrenia, depression, and so on.

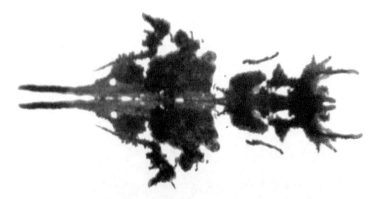

Figure 13-1　Inkblots Used in Rorschach Test
(Inkblots like this one are presented on 10 cards in the Rorschach Test. The patient describes images that he or she sees in the blots.)

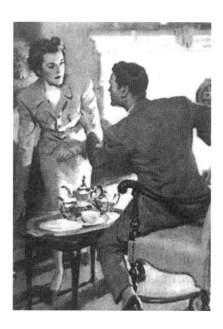

Figure 13-2 A Sample Picture from the Thematic Apperception Test
(The patient is asked to tell the story that the picture illustrates.)

PSYCHIATRIC CLINICAL SYMPTOMS

The following terms describe abnormalities that are evident to an examining mental health professional. Familiarity with these terms will help you understand the next section, "Psychiatric Disorders" (Table 13-1).

Amnesia	Loss of memory.
Anxiety	Varying degrees of uneasiness, apprehension, or dread often accompanied by palpitations, tightness in the chest, breathlessness, and choking sensations.
Apathy	Absence of emotions; lack of interest, emotional involvement, or motivation.
Compulsion	Uncontrollable urge to perform an act repeatedly in an attempt to reduce anxiety.
Conversion	Anxiety becomes a bodily symptom, such as blindness, deafness, or paralysis, that does not have a physical basis.
Delusion	Fixed, false belief that cannot be changed by logical reasoning or evidence.
Dissociation	Uncomfortable thoughts are split off from the person's conscious awareness to avoid mental distress. In extreme cases, dissociation can lead to multiple personalities.
Dysphoria	Intense feelings of depression, discontent, and generalized dissatisfaction with life.
Euphoria	Intense feelings of well-being, elation, happiness, excitement, and joy.
Hallucination	False or unreal sensory perception as, for example, hearing voices when none are present. An illusion is a misperception of an actual sensory stimulus, such as hearing voices in the sound of rustling leaves.

Labile	Variable; undergoing rapid emotional change.
Mania	Elevated, expansive state with talkativeness, hyperactivity, and racing thoughts.
Mutism	No, or very little, ability to speak.
Obsession	Involuntary, persistent idea or emotion; the suffix-mania indicates a strong obsession with something (e.g., pyromania is an obsession with fire).
Paranoia	Overly suspicious system of thinking; fixed delusion that one is being harassed, persecuted, or unfairly treated.

Table 13-1　Psychiatric Disorders

CATEGORY	EXAMPLE(S)		
Anxiety disorders	· Panic disorder · Phobic disorders · Obsessive-compulsive disorder	· Post-traumatic stress disorder · Generalized anxiety disorder	
Bipolar disorders	· Bipolar I · Bipolar II · Cyclothymic disorder		
Depressive disorders	· Major depressive disorder · Persistent depressive disorder (dysthymia) · Seasonal affective disorder (SAD)		
Dissociative disorders	· Identity disorder · Dissociative amnesia · Depersonalization/Derealization disorder		
Eating disorders	· Anorexia nervosa · Bulimia nervosa		
Neurocognitive disorders	· Delirium · Dementia		
Neurodevelopmental disorders	· Intellectual disability disorders · Communication disorders	· Autistic spectrum disorder · Attention-deficit/hyperactivity disorder	
Personality disorders	Cluster A: · Paranoid · Schizoid · Schizotypal	Cluster B: · Antisocial · Borderline · Histrionic · Narcissistic	Cluster C: · Avoidant · Dependent · Obsessive-compulsive
Schizophrenia spectrum and other psychotic disorders (Key features: Delusions, Hallucinations)	· Disorganized thinking (speech) · Abnormal motor behavior · Negative symptoms		
Sexual dysfunctions, paraphilias, and gender dysphoria disorders	· Delayed or premature ejaculation/orgasmic disorders · Exhibitionism · Voyeurism		

CATEGORY	EXAMPLE(S)		continued
Somatic symptom disorders	· Conversion disorder · Illness anxiety disorder		
Substance-related and addictive disorders	Use/Abuse of: · Alcohol · Cannabis · Hallucinogens · Sedatives	· Amphetamines · Cocaine · Opioids	

THERAPEUTIC MODALITIES

Some major therapeutic techniques that are used to treat psychiatric disorders are **psychotherapy**, **electroconvulsive therapy (ECT)**, and **drug therapy (psychopharmacology)**.

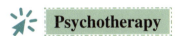

Psychotherapy

Psychotherapy is the treatment of emotional problems and disorders using psychological techniques. The following are psychotherapeutic techniques used by psychiatrists, psychologists, and other mental health professionals.

1. Cognitive-behavioral Therapy (CBT)

This is a relatively short-term, focused psychotherapy for a wide range of psychological problems, including depression, anxiety, anger, marital conflict, fears, and substance abuse.

2. Family Therapy

Treatment of an entire family can help the individual members resolve and understand their conflicts and problems.

3. Group Therapy

In a group with a mental health professional leader as a neutral moderator, patients with similar problems gain insight into their own personalities through discussions and interaction with each other.

4. Hypnosis

A trance (state of altered consciousness) is created to help in recovery of deeply pressed memories. Hypnotic techniques also are used for anxiety reduction, for creating a sense of psychological safety, and for problem solving.

5. Insight-Oriented Psychotherapy

This type of psychotherapy uses face-to-face discussion of life problems and associated feelings. The aim is to increase understanding of underlying conflicts, themes, thoughts, and behavior patterns to improve mood (depressive feelings).

6. Play Therapy

In this form of therapy, the child uses play with toys to express conflicts and feelings that he or she is unable to communicate in a direct manner.

7. Psychoanalysis

This long-term and intense form of psychotherapy seeks to influence behavior and resolve internal conflicts by allowing patients to bring their unconscious emotions to the surface.

8. Sex Therapy

This form of therapy can help people overcome sexual dysfunctions such as frigidity (inhibited sexual response in women), impotence (inability of a man to achieve and/or maintain an erection), and premature ejaculation (release of semen before coitus can be achieved).

9. Supportive Psychotherapy

The therapist offers encouragement, support, and hope to patients facing difficult life transitions and events.

Electroconvulsive Therapy

In **electroconvulsive therapy** (**ECT**), an electrical current is applied to the brain (usually to one hemisphere) after the patient is anesthetized, with assisted ventilation, and given a very short-acting muscle paralytic agent. Actual physical convulsions are therefore imperceptible. This therapy is used chiefly for serious depression and the depressive phase of bipolar (manic-depressive) disorder. ECT is a particularly effective treatment for psychotic depression and can be life-saving when a rapid response is needed.

Drug Therapy

The following are categories of drugs used to treat psychiatric disorders.

1. Antianxiety and antipanic agents

These drugs lessen anxiety, tension, and agitation, especially when they are associated with panic attacks.

2. Antidepressants

These drugs gradually reverse depressive symptoms and return the patient to a more even state, with less persistent and less severe depressive symptoms.

3. Anti-obsessive-compulsive disorder (OCD) agents

These drugs are prescribed to relieve the symptoms of OCD. Tricyclic antidepressants and SSRIs are examples of these agents.

4. Antipsychotics (neuroleptics)

These drugs suppress psychotic symptoms and behavior.

5. Mood stabilizers

These drugs are used primarily to treat patients with the mood changes associated with bipolar disorder.

6. Hypnotics

These drugs are used to produce sleep and relieve insomnia. Examples are sedatives and benzodiazepines.

7. Stimulants

These drugs (amphetamines) are prescribed for attention-deficit/hyperactivity disorder in children and, to a lesser extent, adults.

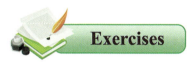

Exercises

I *Match the psychiatric symptoms with their definitions/descriptions that follow.*

amnesia	conversion	mania
anxiety	delusion	mutism
apathy	dissociation	obsession
compulsion	hallucination	

1. nonreactive state marked by inability to speak: _____
2. state of excessive excitability; agitation: _____
3. loss of memory: _____
4. uncontrollable urge to perform an act repeatedly: _____
5. persistent idea, emotion, or urge: _____
6. feelings of apprehension, uneasiness, dread: _____
7. uncomfortable feelings are separated from their real object and redirected toward a second object or behavior pattern: _____
8. anxiety becomes a bodily symptom that has no organic basis: _____
9. absence of emotions; lack of motivation or emotional involvement: _____
10. fixed false belief that cannot be changed by logical reasoning or evidence: _____
11. false or unreal sensory perception: _____

II *Select from the list of psychiatric conditions to complete the sentences that follow.*

anxiety disorders	eating disorders	somatic symptom disorders
delirium	bipolar disorders	substance-related and addictive disorders
dementia	personality disorders	
dissociative disorders	sexual dysfunctions	

1. Disturbances of memory and identity that hide the anxiety of unconscious conflicts are _____.
2. Troubled feelings, unpleasant tension, distress, and avoidance behavior describe a/an _____.

3. Conditions related to regular use of drugs and alcohol are _____.

4. Bulimia and anorexia nervosa are examples of _____.

5. A disorder involving paraphilias is a/an _____.

6. Disorders marked by alternating periods of mania and depression are _____.

7. Mental conditions in which physical symptoms cannot be explained by an actual physical disorder or injury are _____.

8. Lifelong patterns of thought and behavior that are inflexible and cause distress, conflict, and impairment of social functioning are _____.

9. Loss of intellectual abilities with impairment of memory, judgment, and reasoning is _____.

10. Confusion in thinking with faulty perceptions and irrational behavior is _____.

III *Describe some major therapeutic techniques that are used to treat psychiatric disorders.*

APPENDIX

1. Roots of the body

Table 1 Roots of Bodily Concepts

Bodily concepts	Greek roots in English	Latin roots in English	Other roots in English
digestion	pepsia	—	—
disease	pathy	—	—
eating	phagia	vory	—

Table 2 Roots of Body Parts and Components
(Internal anatomy, external anatomy, body fluids, body substances)

Body parts or components	Greek roots	Latin roots	Other roots
abdomen	lapar	abdomin	—
aorta	aort(o)	aort(o)	—
arm	brachi	arm	—
armpit	maschal	axill	—
artery	arteri	—	—
back	not	dors	—
big toe	—	allic, hallic	—
bladder	cyst	vesic	—
blood	haemat, hemat (haem, hem)	sangui, sanguin	—
blood clot	thromb	—	—
blood vessel	angi	vas, vascul	—
body	somat, som	corpor	—
bone	oste	ossi	—
marrow	myel	medull	—
brain	encephal(o)	cerebr	—
breast	mast	mamm(o)	—
chest	steth	pector	—
cheek	parei	bucc	—
ear	ot(o)	aur(i)	—
eggs, ova	oo	ov	—

			continued
Body parts or components	Greek roots	Latin roots	Other roots
eye	ophthalm(o)	ocul(o)	optic(o) (French)
eyelid	blephar(o)	cili, palpebr	—
face	prosop(o)	faci(o)	—
fallopian tubes	salping(o)	—	—
fat, fatty tissue	lip(o)	adip	—
finger	dactyl(o)	digit	—
forehead	—	front(o)	—
gallbladder	cholecyst(o)	fell	—
genitals, sexually undifferentiated	gon(o), phall(o)	—	—
gland	aden(o)	—	—
glans penis or clitoridis	balan(o)	—	—
gums	—	gingiv	—
hair	trich(o)	capill	—
hand	cheir(o), chir(o)	manu	—
head	cephal(o)	capit(o)	—
heart	cardi(o)	cordi	—
hip, hip joint	—	cox	—
horn	cerat(o)	cornu	—
intestine	enter(o)	—	—
jaw	gnath(o)	—	—
kidney	nephr(o)	ren	—
knee	gon	genu	—
lip	cheil(o), chil(o)	labi(o)	—
liver	hepat(o), hepatic	jecor	—
loins, pubic region	episi(o)	pudend	—
lungs	pneumon	pulmon(i), (pulmo)	—
mind	psych	ment	—
mouth	stomat(o)	or	—
muscle	my(o)	—	—
nail	onych(o)	ungui	—
navel	omphal(o)	umbilic	—
neck	trachel(o)	cervic	—

APPENDIX 145

continued

Body parts or components	Greek roots	Latin roots	Other roots
nerve, the nervous system	neur(o)	nerv	—
nipple, teat	thele	papill, mammill	—
nose	rhin(o)	nas	—
ovary	oophor(o)	ovari(o)	—
pelvis	pyel(o)	pelv(i)	—
penis	pe(o)	—	—
pupil (of the eye)	cor, core, coro	—	—
rib	pleur(o)	cost(o)	—
rib cage	thorac(i), thorac(o)	—	—
shoulder	om(o)	humer(o)	—
sinus	—	sinus	—
skin	dermat(o), (derm)	cut, cuticul	—
skull	crani(o)	—	—
stomach	gastr(o)	ventr(o)	—
testis	orchi(o), orchid(o)	—	—
throat (upper throat cavity)	pharyng(o)	—	—
throat (lower throat cavity/voice box)	laryng(o)	—	—
thumb	—	pollic	—
tooth	odont(o)	dent(i)	—
tongue	gloss, glott	lingu(a)	—
toe	dactyl(o)	digit	—
tumour	cel, onc(o)	tum	—
ureter	ureter(o)	ureter(o)	—
urethra	urethr(o), urethr(a)	urethr(o), urethr(a)	—
urine, urinary system	ur(o)	urin(o)	—
uterine tubes	salping(o)	salping(o)	—
uterus	hyster(o), metr(o)	uter(o)	—
vagina	colp(o)	vagin	—
vein	phleb(o)	ven	—
vulva	episi(o)	vulv	—
womb	hyster(o), metr(o)	uter(o)	—
wrist	carp(o)	carp(o)	—

2. List of Affixes

A

Affixes	Meaning	Examples
abdo-min-	of or relating to the abdomen	abdomen, abdominal
acanth-	thorn or spine	acanthion, acanthocyte, acanthoma, acanthulus
acou-	of or relating to hearing	acoumeter, acoustician, hyperacusis
-acusis	hearing	paracusis
aden-	of or relating to a gland	adenocarcinoma, adenology, adenotome, adenotyphus
adip-	of or relating to fat or fatty tissue	adipocyte
aesthesi-	sensation	anesthesia
-al	pertaining to	abdominal, femoral
alb-	denoting a white or pale color	albino
alge(si)-	pain	analgesic
-algia, alg(i)o-	pain	myalgia
ambi-	denoting something as positioned on both sides; describing both of two sides	ambidextrous
amni-	pertaining to the membranous fetal sac (amnion)	amniocentesis
amph(i)-	on both sides	amphicrania, amphismela, amphomycin
amylo-	starchy, carbohydrate-related	amylase, amylophagia
ana-	back, again, up	anaplasia
an-	anus	anal
andr-	pertaining to a man	android, andrology, androgen
angi-	blood vessel	angiogram, angioplasty
ankyl-, ancyl-	denoting something as crooked or bent	ankylosis
ante-	describing something as positioned in front of another thing	antepartum
apo-	away, separated from, derived from	apoptosis
arsen(o)-	of or pertaining to a male; masculine	arsenoblast
arteri(o)-	of or pertaining to an artery	arteriole, artery
arthr-	of or pertaining to the joints, limbs	arthritis
articul-	joint	articulationlactase
-asthenia	weakness	myasthenia gravis
atel(o)-	imperfect or incomplete development	atelocardia
ather-	fatty deposit, soft gruel-like deposit	atherosclerosis
atri-	an atrium (esp. heart atrium)	atrioventricular
aur-	of or pertaining to the ear	aural
axill-	of or pertaining to the armpit (uncommon as a prefix)	axilla
azo(to)-	nitrogenous compound	azothermia

B

Affixes	Meaning	Examples
bacillus	rod-shaped	bacillus anthracis
bacteri-	pertaining to bacteria	bacteriophage, bactericide
blast-	germ or bud	blastomere
blephar(o)-	of or pertaining to the eyelid	blepharoplasty
brachi(o)-	of or relating to the arm	brachium of inferior colliculus
brachy-	indicating "short" or less commonly "little"	brachycephalic
brady-	slow	bradycardia
bronch(i)-	of or relating to the bronchus	bronchitis, bronchiolitis obliterans
bucc(o)-	of or pertaining to the cheek	buccolabial
burs(o)-	bursa (fluid sac between the bones)	bursa, bursitis

C

Affixes	Meaning	Examples
capit-	pertaining to the head (as a whole)	capitation
carcin-	cancer	carcinoma
cardi-	of or pertaining to the heart	cardiology
carp-	of or pertaining to the wrist	carpopedal spasm
-cele	pouching, hernia	hydrocele, varicocele
-centesis	surgical puncture for aspiration	amniocentesis
cephal(o)-	of or pertaining to the head (as a whole)	cephalalgia, hydrocephalus
cerat(o)-	of or pertaining to the cornu; a horn	ceratoid
cerebell(o)-	of or pertaining to the cerebellum	cerebellum
cerebr-	of or pertaining to the brain	cerebrology
cervic-	of or pertaining to the neck, the cervix	cervicodorsal
cheil-	of or pertaining to the lips	angular cheilitis
chem-	chemistry, drug	chemotherapy
chir-, cheir-	of or pertaining to the hand	chiropractor
chol(e)-	of or pertaining to bile	cholaemia (UK)/cholemia (US), cholecystitis
cholecyst(o)-	of or pertaining to the gallbladder	cholecystectomy
chondr(i)o-	cartilage, gristle, granule, granular	chondrocalcinosis
-cidal, -cide	killing, destroying	bacteriocidal
cili-	of or pertaining to the cilia, the eyelashes; eyelids	ciliary
circum-	denoting something as "around" another	circumcision
-clast	break	osteoclast
clostr-	spindle	clostridium
co-	with, together, in association	coenzymes
-coccus	round, spherical	streptococcus

Affixes	Meaning	Examples
col-, colo-, colono-	colon	colonoscopy
colp(o)-	of or pertaining to the vagina	colposcopy
cor-	of or pertaining to eye's pupil	corectomy
cord-	of or pertaining to the heart (uncommon as a prefix)	commotio cordis
cornu-	applied to processes and parts of the body describing them likened or similar to horns	greater cornu
coron(o)-	pertaining to heart	coronary heart disease
cortic(o)	cortex, or outer region	corticosteroid
cost-	of or pertaining to the ribs	costochondral
cox-	of or relating to the hip, haunch, or hip-joint	coxopodite
crani(o)-	belonging or relating to the cranium	craniology
-crine, -crin(o)	to secrete	endocrine
cycl-	circle, cycle	cyclosis
cyph(o)-	denotes something as bent (uncommon as a prefix)	cyphosis
cyst(o)-, cyst(i)-	of or pertaining to the urinary bladder	cystotomy
cyt(o)-, -cyte	cell	cytokine, leukocyte

D

Affixes	Meaning	Examples
dacry(o)-	of or pertaining to tears	dacryoadenitis, dacryocystitis
dactyl(o)-, -dactyl(o)	of or pertaining to a finger, toe	dactylology, polydactyly
dermat(o)-, -derm(o)-	of or pertaining to the skin	dermatology, epidermis, hypodermic, xeroderma
-desis	binding	arthrodesis
dextr(o)-	right, on the right side	dextrocardia
digit-	of or pertaining to the finger (rare as a root)	digit
-dipsia	suffix meaning "(condition of) thirst"	hydroadipsia, oligodipsia, polydipsia
dors(o)-, dors(i)-	of or pertaining to the back	dorsal, dorsocephalad
dromo-	running, conduction, course	dromotropic
duodeno-	duodenum, twelve: upper part of the small intestine (twelve inches long on average), connects to the stomach	duodenal atresia
dynam(o)-	force, energy, power	hand strength dynamometer
-dynia	pain	vulvodynia
dys-	bad, difficult, defective, abnormal	dysentery, dysphagia, dysphasia

E

Affixes	Meaning	Examples
-ectasia, -ectasis	expansion, dilation	bronchiectasis, telangiectasia
-ectomy	denotes a surgical operation or removal of a body part, resection, excision	mastectomy
-emesis	vomiting condition	hematemesis
-emia	blood condition (AmE)	anemia
encephal(o)-	of or pertaining to the brain (Also see cerebro)	encephalogram
episi(o)-	of or pertaining to the pubic region, the loins	episiotomy
-esophageal, esophago-	gullet (AmE)	esophagus
esthesio-	sensation (AmE)	esthesioneuroblastoma, esthesia

F

Affixes	Meaning	Examples
faci-	of or pertaining to the face	facioplegia
fibr-	fiber	fibril, fibrin, fibrinous pericarditis, fibroblast
fil-	fine, hair-like	filament, filum terminale
foramen	hole, opening, or aperture, particularly in bone	foramen magnum
front-	of or pertaining to the forehead	frontonasal

G

Affixes	Meaning	Examples
gastr(o)-	of or pertaining to the stomach	gastric bypass
genu-	of or pertaining to the knee	genu valgum
-geusia	taste	ageusia, dysgeusia, hypergeusia, hypogeusia, parageusia
gingiv-	of or pertaining to the gums	gingivitis
gloss(o)-, glott(o)-	of or pertaining to the tongue	glossology
gnath(o)-	of or pertaining to the jaw	gnathodynamometer
-gnosis	knowledge	diagnosis, prognosis
gon(o)-	seed, semen; also, reproductive	gonorrhea
gyno-, gynaeco- (BrE), gyneco- (AmE)	woman	gynecomastia

H

Affixes	Meaning	Examples
halluc-	to wander in mind	hallucinosis
hemat-, haemato- (haem-, hem-)	of or pertaining to blood	hematology (older form haematology)
hema-, hemo-	blood (AmE)	hemal, hemoglobin

Affixes	Meaning	Examples
hemangi-, hemangio-	blood vessels	hemangioma
hepat- (hepatic-)	of or pertaining to the liver	hepatology, hepatitis
heter(o)-	denotes something as "the other" (of two), as an addition, or different	heterogeneous
hidr(o)-	sweat	hyperhidrosis
hist(o)-, histio-	tissue	histology
humer(o)-	of or pertaining to the shoulder [or (rarely) the upper arm]	humerus
hyster(o)-	of or pertaining to the womb, the uterus	hysterectomy, hysteria

I

Affixes	Meaning	Examples
iatr(o)-	of or pertaining to medicine, or a physician (uncommon as a prefix; common as a suffix, see -iatry)	iatrochemistry
-iatry	denotes a field in medicine of a certain body component	podiatry, psychiatry
ileo-	ileum	ileocecal valve
irid(o)-	iris	iridectomy
isch-	restriction	ischemia
ischio-	of or pertaining to the ischium, the hip joint	ischioanal fossa
-ism	condition, disease	dwarfism
-ismus	spasm, contraction	hemiballismus
-itis	inflammation	tonsillitis
-ium	structure, tissue	pericardium

K

Affixes	Meaning	Examples
kal-	potassium	hyperkalemia
kary-	nucleus	eukaryote
kerat-	cornea (eye or skin)	keratoscope
kine-	movement	akinetopsia, kinesthesia
kyph-	humped	kyphoscoliosis

L

Affixes	Meaning	Examples
labi-	of or pertaining to the lip	labiodental
lapar(o)-	of or pertaining to the abdominal wall, flank	laparotomy
laryng(o)-	of or pertaining to the larynx, the lower throat cavity where the voice box is	larynx

Affixes	Meaning	Examples
-lepsis, -lepsy	attack, seizure	epilepsy, narcolepsy
lingu(a)-, lingu(o)-	of or pertaining to the tongue	linguistics
lip(o)-	fat	liposuction
lith(o)-	stone, calculus	lithotripsy
log(o)-	speech	dialog, catalog, logos
lumb(o)-, lumb(a)-	of or relating to the part of the trunk between the lowest ribs and the pelvis	lumbar vertebrae
lymph(o)-	lymph	lymphedema

M

Affixes	Meaning	Examples
-malacia	softening	osteomalacia
mamm(o)-	of or pertaining to the breast	mammogram
mammill(o)-	of or pertaining to the nipple	mammillaplasty, mammillitis
manu-	of or pertaining to the hand	manufacture
mast(o)-	of or pertaining to the breast	mastectomy
mening(o)-	membrane	meningitis
men-	month, menstrual cycle	menopause, menorrhagia
metr-	pertaining to conditions or instruments of the uterus	metrorrhagia
muscul(o)-	muscle	musculoskeletal system
my(o)-	of or relating to muscle	myoblast
myc(o)-	fungus	onychomycosis
myel(o)-	of or relating to bone marrow or spinal cord	myeloblast
myl(o)-	of or relating to molar teeth or lower jaw	mylohyoid nerve
myring(o)-	eardrum	myringotomy
myx(o)-	mucus	myxoma

N

Affixes	Meaning	Examples
narc(o)-	numb, sleep	narcolepsy
nas(o)-	of or pertaining to the nose	nasal
nephr(o)-	of or pertaining to the kidney	nephrology
nerv-	of or pertaining to nerves and the nervous system (uncommon as a root; neuro- mostly always used)	nerve, nervous system
neur(i)-, neur(o)-	of or pertaining to nerves and the nervous system	neurofibromatosis
noci-	pain, injury, hurt	nociception

O

Affixes	Meaning	Examples
ocul(o)-	of or pertaining to the eye	oculist
odont(o)-	of or pertaining to teeth	orthodontist
odyn(o)-	pain	stomatodynia
-oesophageal, oesophago- (BrE)	oesophagus	
om(o)-	shoulder	omoplate
-oma (singular), -omata (plural)	tumor, mass, fluid collection	sarcoma, teratoma, mesothelioma
omphal(o)-	of or pertaining to the navel, the umbilicus	omphalotomy
onco-	tumor, bulk, volume	oncology
onych(o)-	of or pertaining to the nail (of a finger or toe)	onychophagy
oo-	of or pertaining to an (egg), a woman's egg, the ovum	oogenesis
oophor(o)-	of or pertaining to the woman's (ovary)	oophorectomy
ophthalm(o)-	of or pertaining to the (eye)	phthalmology
-opsy	examination or inspection	biopsy, autopsy
optic(o)-	of or relating to chemical properties of the eye	opticochemical, biopsy
or(o)-	of or pertaining to the mouth	oral
orchi(o)-, orchid(o)-, orch(o)-	testis	orchiectomy, orchidectomy
osse-	bony	osseous
ossi-	bone	peripheral ossifying fibroma
ost(e)-, oste(o)-	bone	osteoporosis, osteoarthritis
ot(o)-	of or pertaining to the ear	otology
ovari(o)-	of or pertaining to the ovaries	ovariectomy
ovo-, ovi-, ov-	of or pertaining to the eggs, the ovum	ovogenesis

P

Affixes	Meaning	Examples
pachy-	thick	pachyderma
palpebr-	of or pertaining to the eyelid (uncommon as a root)	palpebra
papill-	of or pertaining to the nipple (of the chest/breast)	papillitis
papul(o)-	indicates papulosity, a small elevation or swelling in the skin, a pimple, swelling	papulation
-paresis	slight paralysis	pathology
-pathy	denotes (with a negative sense) a disease, or disorder	sociopathy, neuropathy
pector-	breast or chest	pectoralgia, pectoriloquy, pectorophony

continued

Affixes	Meaning	Examples
ped-, -ped-, -pes	of or pertaining to the foot; -footed	pedoscope
ped-, pedo-	of or pertaining to the child	pediatrics, pedophilia
pelv(i)-, pelv(o)-	hip bone	pelvis
-pepsia	denotes something relating to digestion, or the digestive tract	dyspepsia
phaco-	lens-shaped	phacolysis, phacometer, phacoscotoma
-phage, -phagia	forms terms denoting conditions relating to eating or ingestion	dysphagia
-phagy	forms nouns that denotes "feeding on" the first element or part of the word	hematophagy
pharmac-	drug, medication	pharmacology
pharyng-	of or pertaining to the pharynx, the upper throat cavity	pharyngitis, pharyngoscopy
phleb-	of or pertaining to the (blood) veins, a vein	phlebography, phlebotomy
-phobia	exaggerated fear, sensitivity, aversion	arachnophobia
phon-	sound	phonograph, symphony
phos-	of or pertaining to light or its chemical properties, now historic and used rarely. See the common root phot- below	phosphene
phot-	of or pertaining to light	photopathy
phren-, phrenic-	the mind	phrenic nerve, schizophrenia
phyt-	to grow	hydrophyte
-plasia	formation, development	achondroplasia
-plasty	surgical repair, reconstruction	rhinoplasty
pleio-	more, excessive, multiple	pleiomorphism
pleur-	of or pertaining to the ribs	pleurogenous
-plexy	stroke or seizure	cataplexy
pne-, pneum-	air, breath, lung	apnea, pneumatology, pneumonocyte, pneumonia
pod-, -pod-, -pus	of or pertaining to the foot, -footed	podiatry
polio-	denoting a grey color	poliomyelitis
poly-	denotes a "plurality" of something	polymyositis
porphyr-	denotes a purple color	porphyroblast
presby-	old age	presbyopia, presbycusis
proct-	anus, rectum	proctology
prosop-	face	prosopagnosia
psor-	itching	psoriasis
psych-	of or pertaining to the mind	psychology, psychiatry
pterygo-	pertaining to a wing	lateral pterygoid plate
-ptosis	falling, drooping, downward placement, prolapse	apoptosis, nephroptosis
pulmon-, pulmo-	of or relating to the lungs	pulmonary

continued

Affixes	Meaning	Examples
py-	pus	pyometra
pyel-	pelvis	pyelonephritis
pylor-	gate	pyloric sphincter
pyr-	fever	antipyretic

R

Affixes	Meaning	Examples
radi-	radiation	radiowave
radic-	referring to the beginning, or the root, of a structure, usually a nerve or a vein	radiculopathy
rect-	rectum	rectal, rectum
ren-	of or pertaining to the kidney	renal
rhabd(o)-	rod shaped, striated	rhabdomyolysis
rhachi(o)-	spine	rachial, rachialgia, rachidian, rachiopathy
rhin(o)-	of or pertaining to the nose	rhinoceros, rhinoplasty
rhod(o)-	denoting a rose-red color	rhodophyte
-rrhage	burst forth	hemorrhage
-rrhagia	rapid flow of blood	menorrhagia
-rrhaphy	surgical suturing	neurorrhaphy
rubr(o)-	of or pertaining to the red nucleus of the brain	rubrospinal
-rupt	break or burst	erupt, Interrupt

S

Affixes	Meaning	Examples
salping(o)-	of or pertaining to tubes, e.g. fallopian tubes	salpingectomy, salpingopharyngeus muscle
sangui-, sanguine-	of or pertaining to blood	sanguine
sarco-	muscular, fleshlike	sarcoma, sarcoidosis
schist(o)-	split, cleft	schistocyte
schiz(o)-	denoting something "split" or "double-sided"	schizophrenia
scler(o)-	hard	scleroderma
-sclerosis	hardening	atherosclerosis, multiple sclerosis
sial(o)-	saliva, salivary gland	sialagogue
sigmoid(o)-	sigmoid, S-shaped curvature	sigmoid colon
sinus-	of or pertaining to the sinus	sinusitis
somn(o)	sleep	insomniac
-spadias	slit, fissure	hypospadias, epispadias
spasmo-	spasm	spasmodic dysphonia

Affixes	Meaning	Examples
sperma-, spermo-, spermato-	semen, spermatozoa	spermatogenesis
splanchn(i)-, splanchn(o)-	viscera	splanchnology
splen(o)-	spleen	splenectomy
spondyl(o)-	of or pertaining to the spine, the vertebra	spondylitis
squamos(o)-	denoting something as "full of scales" or "scaly"	squamous cell
-stenosis	abnormal narrowing in a blood vessel or other tubular organ or structure	restenosis, stenosis
steth-	of or pertaining to the upper chest, chest, the area above the breast and under the neck	stethoscope
stom-, stomat-	of or pertaining to the mouth; an artificially created opening	stomatogastric, stomatognathic system

T

Affixes	Meaning	Examples
tachy-	denoting something as fast, irregularly fast	tachycardia
-tension, -tensive	pressure	hypertension
tetan-	rigid, tense	tetanus
thely-	denoting something as "relating to a woman, feminine"	thelygenous
therap-	treatment	therapy, therapeutic
therm(o)-	heat	hypothermia
thorac(i)-, thorac(o)-, thoracico-	of or pertaining to the upper chest, chest; the area above the breast and under the neck	thoracic, thorax
thromb(o)-	of or relating to a blood clot, clotting of blood	thrombus, thrombocytopenia
thyr(o)-	thyroid	thyroid
thym-	emotions	dysthymia
-tomy	act of cutting; incising, incision	gastrotomy
ton-	tone, tension, pressure	tone
top(o)-	place, topical	topical anesthetic
tort(i)-	twisted	torticollis
tox(i)-, tox(o)-, toxic(o)-	toxin, poison	toxoplasmosis
trache(a)-	trachea	tracheotomy
trachel(o)-	of or pertaining to the neck	tracheloplasty
trans-	denoting something as moving or situated across or through	transfusion
tri-	three	triangle, triceps

Affixes	Meaning	Examples
trich(i)-, trichia, trich(o)-	of or pertaining to hair, hair-like structure	trichocyst
-tripsy	crushing	lithotripsy
-trophy	nourishment, development	seudohypertrophy
tympan(o)-	eardrum	tympanocentesis

U

Affixes	Meaning	Examples
umbilic-	of or pertaining to the navel, the umbilicus	umbilical
ungui-	of or pertaining to the nail, a claw	unguiform, ungual
ur-	of or pertaining to urine, the urinary system	uraemia/uremia, uremic, ureter, urethra, urology
urin-	of or pertaining to urine, the urinary system	uriniferous
uter(o)-	of or pertaining to the uterus or womb	uterus

V

Affixes	Meaning	Examples
vagin-	of or pertaining to the vagina	vagina
varic(o)-	swollen or twisted vein	varicose
vas(o)-	duct, blood vessel	vasoconstriction
ven-	of or pertaining to the veins, venous blood, and the vascular system	venule, venospasm
ventr(o)-	of or pertaining to the belly; the stomach cavities	ventrodorsal
ventricul(o)-	of or pertaining to the ventricles; any hollow region inside an organ	cardiac ventriculography
vesic(o)-	of or pertaining to the bladder	vesical arteries
viscer(o)-	of or pertaining to the internal organs, the viscera	viscera